Table of Contents

Introduction: Turtle Power: A Shell for Success: Why and How Mindfulness Can Naturally Address ADHD Symptoms and Protect Families

"There is hope, even when your brain tells you there isn't."

— John Green, Turtles All the Way Down

Like a turtle's protective shell, as embodied by John Green's above quote, our brains proactively protect our holistic health and wellness in numerous ways. Yet when our brains do not feel balanced and/or fully understood, we can frequently suffer immensely in so many aspects of our lives as far as socioemotional wellbeing, relationship management, spiritual focus, physical health, psychological wellness, mental stability, financial aptitude, vocational and career success, etc. We can also lose hope, succumb to illnesses, suffer from anxiety, disordered eating, PTSD, OCD, depression, and shatter our self-esteem from this type of detrimental domino effect, if our turtle *shells* are not intact. No, I am not talking about the Teenage Mutant Ninja characters, either, if your child is an avid fan of the movies.

Speaking of shells, how do you protect yourself and kids from ADHD's triggers and outcomes? Have you taught yourself how to wear a mindful *shell* to protect your sanity when parenting kids, tweens, and teens with ADHD? Are you positively and mindfully modeling for your kids how to develop one for their own self-protection, behavioral regulation, sense of advocacy, self-esteem, positive academic and vocational development, and socioemotional growth? Is your children constantly struggling with social relationships, typically sent to the office weekly, lacking academic concentration in school or in the workplace, experiencing behavioral conflicts with peers or family member, and suffering from insomnia or other health ailments? Do you feel like your teenager with ADHD will never learn to drive a car because of his or her inability to focus or self-regulate? Is your tween with ADHD unable to sit through a family meal successfully, both at home and in public, without tapping on the table or constantly getting up from one's chair to roam around the dining room or kitchen? My daughter struggles to remain seated during meals because of her ADHD, so I have full empathy with you. These perky, hissing symptoms denote merely just a few of ADHD's daily challenges, much like a cold-hearted snake in the grass, that we need to tame and train.

However, this book will not discuss reptiles or animal species, but I will offer you a tough and tenacious *turtle shell against ADHD* by delivering evidence-based resources, classroom techniques, psychological tools, parental testimonies from the trenches, tips, and relevant references to guide you to becoming a more mindful parent, family member, coach, mentor, or professional in the exciting but arduous road trip of raising and dealing with a child, tween, or teen with ADHD in mindful, positive, and holistic ways.

If you are a teacher, grandparent, family member, coach, neighbor, or mentor for anyone with ADHD, this book can increase your confidence and lower your stress levels when coping with ADHD. You do not have to feel like you are battling alone.

Firstly, I will briefly discuss what ADHD is and how it can hinder one's holistic health and happiness, if it's not managed properly and positively. Without too much medical mumbo jumbo, I will also uncover typical ADHD myths and stigmas to educate you to see beyond the lingo and labels; let us move toward embracing the strengths that your precious children possess, despite the daunting diagnostic implications.

Moving ahead, I will not move mountains, but I will realistically present mindfulness as an evidence-based practice to address ADHD holistically and also dispel any stereotypes about what mindfulness is not along our literary journey together. Think of this text as a workbook, so you can modify ideas to accommodate your kids' needs.

Once I have given you the *GPS of mindfulness*, you can freely embark on a road trip of love, laughter, knowledge, and resources to cruise and cope with ADHD as a happy, healthy, and peaceful family. I will also show how mindfulness strategies can boost focus, increase self-regulation, enrich social and academic successes, strengthen relationships at home, school, jobs, and community, enhance communication skills, address physical, mental, and spiritual health, as well as instill resilience. Please note that nearly all strategies can be used interchangeably, despite their chapter titles. What I truly find so wonderful about mindfulness is that it can be tailored specifically to your child's ages, needs, lifestyles, strengths, challenges, triggers, etc. It also depends on your parenting style and preferences, so it is all about you the adult, too!

Plus, I will also explore essential m*ood foods* and other holistic nutritional tips to manage ADHD within your homes using a more *back to the basics* approach. What family doesn't like to eat or snack during a road trip, right?

With this deep hunger and thirst for knowledge on the brain, let us delve into this book's main objectives, so you can take back your family's life, health, peace, and happiness if ADHD has been zapping your joy, sanity, wellness, and unity lately.

As a result of this book, readers will be able to...

- Understand what ADHD is and how it simultaneously impacts the brain, behaviors, social relationships, physical functioning, communicative aptitude, mental health, academic progress, and vocational readiness and success.
- Explore the various holistic challenges of parenting, coaching, teaching, and raising kids, tweens, and teens with ADHD and your own adult role in this process.
- Recognize the overlapping consequences upon families when failing to employ mindfulness into daily routines and parenting paradigms.
- Identify and dispel common ADHD stigmas, stereotypes, fallacies, and myths that often prevent our kids and families from excelling.
- Summarize what mindfulness entails using critical research, personal examples with my own children, and former classroom testimonies to further validate the book's contents.
- Clarify what mindfulness is not as far as stereotypes and mainstream misconceptions.
- Overview mindfulness (MAPS) for ADHD, research and resources to validate its main ideas, and its array of holistic benefits.
- Suggest practical ways to employ mindfulness daily at home to increase kids' sense of focus and self-regulation aptitude.
- Deliver practical, creative, mindful, and age appropriate strategies to utilize and modify mindfulness to better enhance kids, social, communicative, academic, and vocational skills.

- List mindfulness tools and tactics for academic success and career readiness to better cope with ADHD.
- Articulate how mindfulness can enrich self-esteem in kids, tweens, and teens with ADHD.
- Link mindfulness with effective communication skills and tactics from pre-K age to 18+ years old.
- Show concretely through many examples how mindfulness can boost physical, spiritual, psychological, social, and behavioral health.
- Discuss practical methods to reduce familial and parental stress from ADHD using a ton of mindfulness techniques.
- Highlight *mood foods* and healthy beverages; depict the back to the basic link and tips for mindfulness eating and holistic dietary management at home.
- Validate how mindfulness can promote better resilience in kids, teens, tweens, adults, and families overall.

Chapter 1: Brain Balance and Finding the Yellow Brick Road: What is ADHD and Its Holistic Challenges for Kids, Tweens, Teens, Parents, and Families?

Can't you give me brains?" asked the Scarecrow.

"You don't need them. You are learning something every day. A baby has brains, but it doesn't know much. Experience is the only thing that brings knowledge, and the longer you are on earth the more experience you are sure to get. "

— L. Frank Baum, The Wonderful Wizard of Oz

How many of you are avid *Wizard of Oz* fans? Well, I, too, love this classic book, *The Wiz*, and its various film versions, but I never really fathomed its deeper wisdom and transformative life lessons until I became a parent later in life in my forties. As a former teacher of at risk teens for over 15 years and proud mama of two daughters, one with an ADHD diagnosis, I now associate the cast of *Wizard of Oz* characters with clear connections to labels like OCD, ADHD, ODD, PTSD, and other mental health diagnoses. Of course my interpretation could be a bit deep (and dark) for such a coveted children's piece, but I want to use this metaphor today to show and inspire you how with love, team work, patience, knowledge, and experience, you, too, can excel on your own *yellow brick road* of parenting, coaching, mentoring, and childrearing, despite the ADHD challenges.

While I do not promise any cures, easy solutions, or *ruby red slippers* in this book, I will earnestly and passionately speak from parental and teaching experiences, coupled with years of psychological and holistic research on side from workshops, professional trainings, self-studies, and so on. Are you ready to journey together to find the *Emerald City* of family peace, enlightenment, academic support, and holistic health in the plight to manage ADHD more naturally?

First of all, I want to begin by exploring what ADHD is. Why is this label tossed around so aimlessly, often in jokes, excuses, learned helplessness, criminal justice cases, and so many other links in society, especially ones that are negative, stigmatizing, and alienating? Well, ADHD stands for Attention Deficit Hyperactivity Disorder, one of the most common childhood disorders that can often persist through adolescence and adulthood. According to an article by Abdolahzadeh, Mashhadi, & Tabibi (2017) in the *Journal of Fundamentals of Mental Health* (http://jfmh.mums.ac.ir/?_action=showPDF&sc=1&article=8214&_ob=b87cb0d7e0077e6a5449f892bł its prevalence is increasing due to all the technological and digital innovations in our world today.

Because each child's symptoms may vary uniquely, Sharpe's (2011) article, "Hyper One Day, Calm the Next," from *Scientific American Mind* specifies how ADHD has three subtypes: hyperactive, inattentive and both combined (p. 10). What does it look like in school, in the car, at the dinner table among your kiddos, students, team members, or family members? People with ADHD often struggle to focus, self-regulate, meet deadlines, complete tasks, and achieve other essential life skills.

Additionally, the same study above further confirms how ADHD is officially defined by the fifth Psychiatric Association's Diagnostic and Statistical Manual (DSM-5) as the sustainable pattern of attention deficit and impulsivity/hyperactivity, which includes coping with attention deficit, hyperactivity, and impulsivity (http://jfmh.mums.ac.ir/?_action=showPDF&sc=1&article=8214&_ob=b87cb0d7e0077e6a5449f892bł Yunus (2019) also insists in *Exceptional Child* how ADHD presently affects approximately "11% of US children aged 4-17. The Centers for Disease Control estimates that 2.7 million children in the U.S. are currently taking medication for ADHD" (p. 24). Like mindfulness, which addresses all the integrated parts of a person as far as social, emotional, cognitive, spiritual, physical, behavioral, and psychological, ADHD is also a multifaceted disorder that must be faced in such a holistic manner. In sum, Yunus (2019) elaborates how ADHD can disrupt "…cognitive, academic, behavioral, emotional and social functioning. It may be associated with other conditions, such as learning disabilities, anxiety, depression and conduct disorders. The cause is unknown and thought to be a combination of genetic and environmental factors" (p. 24).

Are any of these descriptors evident among your own kiddos, tweens, or teens presently? My oldest daughter has the wiggles, waggles, and fidgets all day and night (and all the times in between) unless I apply some of these mindfulness tactics to the rescue!

Along the same lines, various studies also confirm how an ADHD brain differs from the typical brain as an ADHD brain has "shown less activity and less volume in certain areas of the ADHD brain—as much as 14 percent less volume in the anterior cingulate cortex (Huff, 2016, p. 3), for example. Kunus (2019) also delineates other typical signs and symptoms, ranging from a host of possible outcomes like inattention, impulsivity, disorganization, forgetfulness, poor con-centration, academic underachievement, inability to follow instructions or finish tasks, risky activities without consideration of consequences, disruptive behaviors, interrupting others, and impatience" (p. 24).

Next, I want to further highlight why ADHD is so prevalent in our current era, as expressed in the early research. Do you ever feel like your brain is on fire, constantly exploding, buzzing, and blitzing from emails, calls, texts, and to-dos that manifest in our modern, manic world? Huff (2016) from the book, *Living Well With ADHD*, warns how we are actually living in such a detrimental time, often called "ADD Nation" and "Butterfly Brain" (p. 3). These butterflies are the beautiful, bubby ones, because we are all at risk of ADHD right now under this supersized, fast-paced mentality and lifestyle.

In brief, our human brains are literally bombarded everyday with overloads of sensations, stimuli, and data without much time to sleep, pause, or breathe. When was the last time you really accrued 8 hours of uninterrupted sleep as a parent, coach, mentor, teacher, nurse, or other professional? As a result of these complex challenges, we must find more natural and back to the basic ways to address ADHD, starting with young children, in particular. Let us seek use this book to set our kids, tweens, and tweens with ADHD on a smoother course for a more mindful mindset for the rest of their lives and careers!

Is there a cure, vaccination, or remedy for ADHD? While there are different treatment methods for treating this disorder, my book will not cover pharmacological ones as my focus here is on mindful, natural, and holistic interventions. Don't worry, though, you do not have to be a devout yogi, vegan, or vegetarian to reap the benefits of mindful parenting, despite many contemporary myths and mainstream misconceptions about this lifestyle. You also do not have to be a *granola guy or gal* to deeply benefit from the simple, natural strategies to succeed against the angst that ADHD can often inflict upon our families, friends, students, and neighbors right now.

Do you recall how Scarecrow's character was literally off kilter because he lacked a brain in the story? Well, kids with ADHD have brains, but their balance is misaligned, which can frequently manifest in various physical, behavioral, linguistic, academic, socioemotional, neuropsychological, and cognitive issues. Kunus (2019) further highlights how ADHD can manifest "as fidgeting, difficulty remaining seated, inability to remain quiet, or restlessness. The disorder is seen more frequently in boys and there seems to be a genetic propensity among siblings with the disorder" (p. 24).

When looking at gender bender implications a bit more in ADHD statistics and research, I also found from Bates (2012) in "Calm Down, Boys" from *Psychology Today* how many clinicians sometimes tend to not recognize the symptoms of ADHD when they appear in females and within teens of both genders. Bates (2012) also presented some fascinating diagnostic discrepancies related to gender by the fact that a boy is usually "twice as likely to be diagnosed with ADHD as a girl with the same symptoms, even if he does not fit all the diagnostic criteria" (p. 17). While my book does not cover "Men Are From Mars; Women Are From Venus" type of gender specific discussions, I seek a more equitable and inclusive way to treat and cope with ADHD in all kids, tweens, and teens.

Along the same lines of challenges when diagnosing ADHD, I admit how it can be tricky in all ages, but especially during adolescence when teenagers both with and without ADHD tend to exude much more erratic, "impulsive, inattentive, and disorganized--but not necessarily hyperactive, explains Margaret Sibley, a psychologist at Florida International University. Different symptoms do not mean fewer problems. A1 6-year-old girl who runs stop signs and can never find her homework might not be a rebel--she could just have ADHD" (Bates, 2012, p. 17). For the sake of equity, this book offers ideas for both genders and also encourages parents of transgender kids with ADHD to try the same techniques. I was a secondary English/Drama educator, dance teacher, and director in many at risk schools, so I also use my life lessons and career insights within this book.

Cyber nod if you feel a bit like the Scarecrow or are raising, teaching, mentoring, or modeling for a child, tween, or teen presently with some of those scattered habits or emotional displays, as noted above? The diagnostic part of ADHD is extremely perplexing, so always enlist the help of teachers, counselors, doctors, psychologists, other professionals, and parents in the ongoing process and always seek ongoing support from your loved ones.

Diagnostically, ADHD can be daunting. According to some findings by Schipani (2008) in "Thriving with ADHD" in *Scholastic Parent & Child*, kids with ADHD often have other conditions that might be missed. "For example, 50 to 80 percent might also have a learning disability. A quarter of ADHD kids also have anxiety issues. About 7 percent have tics" (p. 68). My book will later focus on the value of keeping food and parental logs about kids' symptoms, strengths, diets, and struggles, so you can share relevant information when you work with others on your kids' teams to cope collaboratively and mindfully with ADHD.

Why and how do I know so much about this sensitive topic? On a personal level, my oldest daughter, for example, has the ADHD diagnosis, which initially caused me some guilt frustration, anger, pain, blame, confusion, shame, anxiety, and depression as a parent. However, just like addressing any special need such as diabetes or asthma, I have learned how to balance and tame her "dragons." She loves the *How to Train Your Dragon* movies, so I have creatively and mindfully taught her that ADHD is similar to dragon training; in turn, this simple analogy has worked wonders for her preschool brain! What simple comparison can you use today to help your kid, tween, or teen not to be discouraged or deflated by one's ADHD diagnosis? Come on, and be creative! Let the dragons roar!

As far as ADHD's holistic challenges, I will also thoroughly explain how ADHD manifests in my own child's home and academic life as well as social behaviors, psychological wellness, physical health, etc. For instance, she has to be verbally told directions at least five times more than my other daughter during simple daily skills. I have to constantly re-direct my daughter to give her autonomy and tools to fan the flames of ADHD because she and I both can become easily frustrated and defensive. Does this type of re-rerun sound familiar in your home, car, soccer field, dance studio, or classroom?

Plus, my daughter with ADHD also benefits tremendously from having recurrent visual cues for daily tasks such as brushing her teeth, remaining seated during mealtimes, washing her hands after using the bathroom, and other basic rituals because her mind is always racing so furiously, like a hurried (yet adorable) little hamster in a wheel. She further struggles with self-regulation and managing her emotions proactively, so I find songs as also quite helpful as well as adding gestures and dance moves, since she is highly kinesthetic and hands-on in her learning style and preferences.

In fact, she is like a tiny tornado in the house, always full of endless energy, and constantly in motion, often bouncing, tapping her toes, twirling her hair, and exhibiting other signs of ADHD. She is also as robust and erratic as a tropical storm if she is not reminded or redirected to take deep belly breaths, get enough sleep eat night, watch candies, and eat properly. Do you have a recurrent case of stormy weather in the parenting, teaching, mentoring, or coaching forecast that has brought you to this book today? Well, put on a pair of rain boots, bust out that umbrella, and let it rain down on us with mindfulness!

Now that you have learned a bit about how I ride the storm and *train dragons* in my mindful mamasita duties and credentials as a teacher, I want to also list some other eminent challenges facing the general population with an ADHD diagnosis. For starters, several of the major challenges of ADHD typically involve emotion dysregulation, poor listening aptitude, and impaired functional domains. Studies by Hoxhaj, Sadohard, Borel, Sobanski, Muller, and Philipsen (2018) in an article from the *European Archives of Psychiatry and Clinical Neuroscience* strongly exclaim how ADHD is also linked to lack of concentration, elevated impulsivity, and even higher rates of depression and anxiety (https://www.ncbi.nlm.nih.gov/pubmed/29356899). What are your most pressing ones observed in kiddos when parenting a child with ADHD, coaching a teen who is restless and always on the move, or tutoring a tween who is always late or combative?

Furthermore, the same preceding study also listed poor academic achievements, higher dropout rates, increased behavioral and attendance problems, at risk for mental and substance use disorders, criminality, and unemployment (https://www.ncbi.nlm.nih.gov/pubmed/29356899) as possible red flags to watch with ADHD, without proper, proactive interventions. Talk about some cases of those evil flying monkeys from the *Wizard of Oz*, right?

However, I want to urge us all to save the labels for the soup cans, okay? Like your own amazing children, students, and team members, my daughter with ADHD is also extremely kind, super artistic, dramatic, intelligent, funny, social, and highly empathetic. She is so much more than a label, an acronym, a diagnosis in a chart, an IEP; and so are your kind kiddos, terrific tweens, and amazing adolescents! We simply have to address them differently as parents, teachers, mentors, and coaches: let us now realize how to align with and accommodate their unique needs and gifts. Are you eager to *melt away more of the mask of ADHD* as we address and rectify some common stigmas and myths in Chapter 2?

Chapter 2: Melting the Mask: Addressing ADHD Stigmas and Myths

"No man, for any considerable period, can wear one face to himself and another to the multitude, without finally getting bewildered as to which may be the true."

— *Nathaniel Hawthorne, The Scarlet Letter*

Now that you have a better idea of what ADHD is and how it can impact holistic health on so many intersecting domains, this chapter investigates how we can *melt away the mask of myths, stigmas, and misconceptions* about ADHD. Just as the Tin Man wore his tough metallic exterior but was so vulnerable and compassionate inside, we must not allow the ADHD *mask* to disguise our children's true talents, dreams, happiness, strengths, skills, and potentials.

In sum, let us address and rectify what I fondly nickname "the Evil 8" common myths, stigmas, and misconceptions surrounding ADHD based on my rich experiences as a parent and secondary educator:

- **Jolly Green Giant**: Like the Jolly Green Giant, who grows his veggies and endless height, many people falsely believe that their children will likely *outgrow* ADHD once he or she enters middle school. Many parents also presume that ADHD is just a phase.

On the contrary, while it is important to again emphasize how each case of ADHD is different, studies from Hoxhaj, Sadohard, Borel, Sobanksi, Muller, and Philipsen (2018) also report how ADHD's estimated prevalence is 2-3% in the adult population (https://www.ncbi.nlm.nih.gov/pubmed/29356899). For this reason, we must not only teach parents and families but also kids how to calmly cope and confidently self advocate because ADHD can potentially follow across the lifespan. ADHD is definitely not merely child's play and studies even estimate that increasing use (and abuse) of technological and digital devices is causing greater incidences among adults. Anyone ready for a tech timeout?

- **Gender Bender:** I am constantly hearing endless and biased excuses that "Boys will be boys" as far as ADHD and that it's strictly applicable to boys. In reality, ADHD does not discriminate as far as gender, socioeconomic class, race, culture, lifestyle, religion, ability, disability, language, religion, etc. Girls can also exhibit ADHD, as my daughter's story demonstrates.

- **Pop a Pill:** How many times have you mentioned this one to a nurse or doctor? There is often a prevalent belief that if my kid takes medication regularly, then his or her ADHD will instantly vanish. Again, this book will not explore pharmacological interventions, so definitely consult with your doctors first and foremost. In my own daughter's case, she does not presently require medication for her ADHD, but many cases medically warrant it.

On the flip side, numerous studies highlight how medication alone cannot usually and wholly "fix" ADHD. In fact, the earlier (2018) finding revealed how "20-50% of ADHD patients are non-responders to medication, have contraindications, or prefer a non-pharmacological treatment. Therefore alternative treatment approaches are needed" (https://www.ncbi.nlm.nih.gov/pubmed/29356899). The aim of this book is to add a natural, holistic approach to complement whatever you are currently doing for your child's ADHD.

- **Candyland:** This stereotype is especially prevalent during Easter, Halloween, and Valentine's Day, right? So many parents merely blame increased sugar intakes on why kids are exuding more ADHD symptoms. Of course there are proven triggers in ADHD, especially related to sugar and all that junk in the trunk, as we'll discuss in chapter 14, ADHD is likely a combination (or smoothie!) of nature and nurture elements.
- **Bored Out of Her/His Gourd**: The blame game is also a frequent claim by many parents for an ADHD diagnosis. We tend to want to blame TV, teachers, genes, diets, peers, and so many other root causes. Many parents often adamantly defend how there is absolutely nothing wrong with their children; instead, some parents allege that teachers are just boring, old school, and/or and do not truly like or fully understand kids, tweens, and teens with ADHD. Have you heard this one before?

Of course there can be school days/daze issues, but most educators honestly have the best intentions and exemplify true professionals in my tenure. While the boredom claims can hold some validity on a case by case basis, research cautions how academic achievement can be greatly hindered due to ADHD. In my own experience as an educator, kids today are especially challenged amid the current pressures of standardized testing, which afford teachers less time, flexibility, and freedom to infuse music, drama, the arts, games, and other creative forms of multiple intelligence and sensory-based activities to target attention issues and memory capacity.

- **Ants in the Pants**: Too many parents swiftly dismiss mindfulness and feel that it is even ludicrous to think that mindfulness might work for a kid with ADHD. Have you ever felt like your kid could never possibly sit still long enough to try yoga or meditation? If mindfulness sounds like a joke to you, then I will integrate some basic examples from my own daughter's journey into mindfulness as well as global research to show how it can address those "ants in the pants" type kiddos and behaviors!

To use a personal testimony, when my daughter is not training her dragons, she is actively involved in sports, music, art, dance, karate, and yoga. I, too, was initially quite skeptical about how a child as young as age 3 could survive a kids' yoga class, but she actually flourished in it at the local recreation center. She even taught me rock pose and a ton of other restorative lessons, so give your kiddos credit and a chance to show mind over matter!

- **Bad Seed:** If Lady Gaga's song, "Born this Way," has become your rationale for ADHD in your child as far as his or her genetic disposition, again, there is the whole nature/nurture debate that we won't delve into today. Yet please do not label your child as a troublemaker, clown, drama queen, future thug, or criminal based on his or her ADHD diagnosis.
- **Sporties for Shorties**: Are you fed up with people suggesting that if you enroll your child with ADHD in sports, dance, or martial arts, then the ADHD will automatically dissipate? Of course movement and exercises of all types are extremely beneficial and also key parts of mindfulness. Chapter 11 will explore some specific physical and

movement-based interventions for you to consider.

Like mentioned in my own daughter's journey, keeping her actively engaged does help to better regulate her ADHD much more than when she is merely sitting around staring at a TV or gadget for hours upon end. However, I want to actively dispel the myth that a few sessions at the YMCA can totally eliminate ADHD. Movements, sports, exercise, dance, and other forms of kinesthetic activation can definitely help to cope and manage ADHD, but a cure is not guaranteed from movement alone.

Chapter 3: Center Stage: What's Mindfulness and Its Brief History

"We resonate with one another's sorrows because we are interconnected. Being whole and simultaneously part of a larger whole, we can change the world simply by changing ourselves. If I become a center of love and kindness in this moment, then in a perhaps small but hardly insignificant way, the world now has a nucleus of love and kindness it lacked the moment before. This benefits me and it benefits others."
— Jon Kabat-Zinn, Wherever You Go, There You Are: Mindfulness Meditation in Everyday Life

Now that you are more aware of what ADHD is and some usual myths, misconceptions, and stigmas surrounding it, let us shine the spotlight on *center stage* as we talk about what mindfulness is and how this approach evolved historically in this chapter. As the above quote suggests, mindfulness is all about centering, connecting with one's self and others, surrounding oneself in love, empathy, and compassion. It also cultivates the power of change that we all possess within each of us. In sum, it is extremely empowering, individualized, affirmative, communal, transformative, and uplifting. So much easier than a parenting cape or magic wand, right?

For all the history buffs out there, I will now briefly trace how, when, and why mindfulness began. While mindfulness, yoga, and meditation were critical features of Eastern philosophies, ways of life, and religions since antiquity, most scholars agree that the Western roots of mindfulness derived from Jon Kabat-Zinn, the founder of the mindfulness movement https://time.com/1556/the-mindful-revolution/).   Pickert (2014) specifically credits Kabat-Zinn as the pioneer for this movement since he devised a curriculum called Mindfulness Based Stress Reduction (MBSR). Developed in 1979, this approach basically aimed to rewire our brains naturally and in an integrated manner. It also focused on how to quiet our minds, slow down our thoughts, sit more in silence, and become more self-aware of what is surrounding us right now within the present moment. Put away the phones, toss aside those shopping lists, and get more mindful with me!

If you are like I am and constantly googling for new songs, games, and parenting techniques, mindfulness offers a one-stop-shop of sorts for free and fun interventions. Your role is less of a police officer as a parent and more of a guide on the side within this approach. Think of it a bit like a movie director but less drama. Also, mindfulness is so much more serene without all the red carpet chaos, Hollywood scandals, and pervasive paparazzi.

Speaking of Hollywood, does your child with ADHD currently have a tendency to be more *center stage* as far as *the center of attention*, rather than centered and balanced? I completely empathize because my daughter with ADHD constantly dons costumes and capes (literally) and loves being the sage on the stage 24/7; besides, she also has highly erratic, dramatic, all or nothing thoughts and actions. It's difficult for her to find a happy medium sense of center and balance among daily routines. However, mindfulness holds the potential to really *center* our kiddos in the calming sense to achieve better holistic balance, happiness, and health.

How does this work? Does the Wizard just appear in a cloud of smoke and make mindfulness poof away all the ADHD despair? No, mindfulness isn't a magic potion, but Poissant, Mendrek, Talbot, Khoury, and Nolan (2019) reveal how Mindfulness-based interventions (MBIs) are becoming increasingly popular right now as treatments for physical and psychological problems   (https://mindfulnessnews.wordpress.com/2019/05/17/behavioral-and-cognitive-impacts-of-mindfulness-based-interventions-on-adults-with-attention-deficit-hyperactivity-disorder-a-systematic-review/) in adolescence through adulthood. Mindfulness is one of today's hottest buzz words, but it is definitely more than just a cool trend or buzz word.

What is more, clinical studies from Siebelink, Bögels, Boerboom, de Waal, Buitelaar, Speckens, & Greven (2018) praise mindfulness as an add-on to care-as-usual in *BMC Psychiatry*. Despite its cool vibes, mindfulness is not just a catchy cliché. Do I have to sport tie-dyed clothing, chant under salt lamps, and feed my kids only green smoothies and kale chips in order to be authentically mindful? No. Just be you!

In sum, mindfulness is often defined simply as the trainable, nonjudgmental path to learn how to pay close attention, foster appreciation, and engage in experiences fully in the present moment (https://www.ncbi.nlm.nih.gov/pubmed/29356899). A good way to remember it is PPN: Purposeful, Present, and Now. With such an easy formula, how can you not try it as part of your parenting paradigm, eh? Now if I could just reminder all of my other PINs and daily passwords!

In addition, scholars also maintain how mindfulness essentially works by tapping into self-regulation through three main processes: enhanced attention control, improved emotional regulation, and better self-awareness/body awareness (https://www.ncbi.nlm.nih.gov/pubmed/29356899). Those are amazing feats for mindfulness as a mighty multitasker! Before mindfulness, my daughter used to complain and lament how she literally couldn't control her little body; likewise, this claim is definitely a legitimate and common one with an ADHD diagnosis.

In essence, mindfulness is cited as advantageous for addressing the following:

- **Brain Games:** Mindfulness can often help to enrich executive cognitive functioning that boosts concentration, working memory, speech, etc. In particular, Poissant, Mendrek, Talbot, Khoury, & Nolan highlight how the use of mindfulness meditation training yielded major improvements in both executive and emotional dysregulation (https://mindfulnessnews.wordpress.com/2019/05/17/behavioral-and-cognitive-impacts-of-mindfulness-based-interventions-on-adults-with-attention-deficit-hyperactivity-disorder-a-systematic-review/) under repeated analysis. It can allow your kids, tweens, and teens with ADHD to stop feeling like their brains are playing games with them.

- **Soul Surfer:** Like a soulful surfer who bravely glides and freely rides the waves, mindfulness will not wholly remove all stress and challenges in life, but it can certainly help kids, tweens, and tweens better manage emotions, cope with stress, achieve a higher quality of life, etc. Aloha to that!

- **School of Rock:** Mindfulness is often praised for *rocking* better focus, grade point averages in school and fewer disciplinary incidents (https://mindfulnessnews.wordpress.com/2019/05/17/behavioral-and-cognitive-impacts-of-mindfulness-based-interventions-on-adults-with-attention-deficit-hyperactivity-disorder-a-systematic-review/). Are you excited to *rock on* with mindfulness?

Chapter 4: Beyond Buzz Words: What Mindfulness is Not

"Imperfections are not inadequacies; they are reminders that we're all in this together."
— Brené Brown

As expressed in Brene Brown's quote, mindfulness allows us to accept and embrace our perfect imperfections in life and within our loved ones. However, like self-care and other current buzz words, mindfulness often gets misconstrued. As far as clarifying further what mindfulness is not, it is not a mind *full* of junk or randomness; it is also not mindlessness. What does this really mean? Recent studies by Kudesia (2019) further elucidate how people are mindless when they "rely primarily on established concepts to interpret situations, which makes them respond to situations without discerning their unique features" (https://journals.aom.org/doi/abs/10.5465/amr.2015.0333). Let us seek to work to see beyond buzz words and trends together as we cope calmly and confidently with ADHD in our lives.

Are you excited to join me now in this chapter as I break down the *Fab 4 Fibs* to reiterate what mindfulness is not in these creative tips?

1. **Men Are from Mars; Women Are From Venus:** Contrary to any fallacies, mindfulness is applicable for men and women, boys and girls. Even aliens for that matter-just saying!
2. **Losing My Religion:** Remember that catchy R.E.M. song from the 90s? Well, mindfulness is not a religion; in fact, it embodies more of a lifestyle or an approach. While it involves some spiritual aspects like meditation, anyone, regardless of religious beliefs or lack thereof, can fully engage in mindfulness. Karaoke, folks?
3. **Pretzel Power:** Mindfulness is not about being skinny, flexible, or holding poses for hours. While yoga can be one way to achieve mindfulness, there are tons of other strategies to try. Stay tune as I will further explain more in upcoming chapters.
4. **OMing Out:** Mindfulness is not the same as meditation, despite the

fact that the two terms are frequently used interchangeably. To clarify, meditation is indeed a form of mindfulness, but they are not 100% synonymous. Sorry, no twins here!

Chapter 5: GPS of ADHD: Overview of Mindfulness (MAPS) And Holistic Benefits

"The present moment is filled with joy and happiness. If you are attentive, you will see it."

— Thich Nhat Hanh, Peace Is Every Step: The Path of Mindfulness in Everyday Life

After reviewing the Fab 4 Fibs about what mindfulness is not, Chapter 5 will cover more about mindfulness, introduce you to MAPS, and cite its various holistic benefits. Like the sentiment in the quote above, mindfulness directs our attention gently and deliberately, offering us peace, joy, and contentment in the process. Are you ready to get your Zen on?

As we cruise down the *yellow brick road* of parenting together, think of mindfulness like Dorothy's loyal companion, Toto, as he faithfully remained present, patient, calm, nonjudgmental, and supportive. Like a *GPS*, mindfulness can direct our thoughts, energy, behaviors, and beliefs in a positive, focused, and clear direction.

What exactly does the MAPs part mean? It does not involve travelling to amazing Australia, gorgeous Greece, or marvelous Madagascar. Instead, it refers to Mindful Awareness Practices (MAPs) that enable us to focus our attention more prominently in the present moment and to develop a non-judgmental, accepting attitude (https://www.ncbi.nlm.nih.gov/pubmed/29356899). Has your child ever been bullied? Well, mindfulness cannot only address ADHD but a host of other issues as well.

This GPS further steers our ability to self-regulate our attention and to identify and deal with negative feelings in a positive, objective manner. We can use MAPs by sitting in silence, deep breathing, visualizing, and other tactics.

In my own parenting experience, I realized that timeouts were utterly meaningless and actually counterproductive for my daughter with ADHD, so I decided to have her "re-charge her batteries" when she required support and help with self-regulation and impulse control. This notion was less punitive than using the words "timeout," so she was instantly less agitated by the term. Accordingly, she now gets to choose a safe, quiet place in the house (or mall, restaurant, grocery store, a relative's home) to engage in deep breathing and relaxing time while I use a timer for her "re-charging" station.

How did mindfulness matter? Just the small changes in language and added breathing prompts have given her much more accountability over her actions. Since she is only 4 (but she acts like she is 24!), I set the timer for 4 minutes to align more with her attention span. I will cover more of these techniques thoroughly in future chapters, especially 6-11.

Does this *GPS* work? Unlike your driving devices that can often lead you astray, MAPS works quite well. For example, research insists that mindfulness-based therapy is useful in reducing clinical symptoms in adolescents with ADHD. Participants were better able to express themselves, reflect and evaluate, and perceive the present time (http://jfmh.mums.ac.ir/?_action=showPDF&sc=1&article=8214&_ob=b87cb0d7e0077e6a5449f892bt You have probably heard the popular expression, "Check yourself before you wreck yourself?" Well, that is basically how this *GPS of MAPS* operates.

In the same study cited above by Abdolahzadeh, Mashhadi, & Tabibi (2017), participants justified these improvements in self-regulation, and they noticed gains specifically in diverse areas such as impulse control, better concentration, and less distractibility overall. Let these statistics motivate you to add a few mindfulness moments to your own parental toolbox today!

Adding to these accolades, other MAPs research also presents some compelling evidence. MAPS also greatly improved emotional regulation among study participants in several teen studies (https://www.ncbi.nlm.nih.gov/pubmed/29356899). Mindfulness meditation was specifically heralded for helping with attentional process concentration and decreasing impulsivity in healthy participants. Even strides in working memory capacity were also mentioned. Since I literally forgot where my car was today in a crowded parking garage, I can certainly use some of these memory tips to keep my own self in check, too. What about you? How can MAPS serve as a wonderful addition to your parenting arsenal of activities?

Chapter 6: Cruise Control Mindfulness for Focus and Self-Regulation

It's calm under the waves in the blue of my oblivion."

— Fiona Apple

How many of your kids are fans of the *Moana* movie? Well, I often allude to the film because it's so wonderful for displaying how we can literally and metaphorically calm waves of stress, anxiety, low self-esteem, and family strife. Check it out if you are seeking a sweet, fun, empowering, diverse, family movie night suggestion. The music from the movie's soundtrack is really cool as well!

As mentioned earlier in the last chapter, self-regulation is one of the major perks of using mindfulness with kids, tweens, or teens. It allows them to place their brains and bodies on *cruise control*. Are you ready to transform your home and kids from chaotic to calm?

Additional reasons to try mindfulness to encourage better focus and increased self-regulation among kids with ADHD reflect compelling studies with elementary students from Keller, Ruthruff, Keller, Hoy, Gaspelin, & Bertolini (2017) in the *Journal of Research in Childhood Education* (https://www.researchgate.net/publication/318919569_Your_Brain_Becomes_Graders_in_a_School-Based_Mindfulness_Intervention). They allege how self-regulation of attention and emotion are vital skills for students to master in order to learn efficiently and cooperate well with others interpersonally. The study praised mindfulness for helping 4th graders not only improve academic scores but also many dimensions of social, behavioral, and emotional growth. The study also depicted how mindfulness helps to achieve greater emotional awareness, "arguably the first step toward regulation, is associated with decreases in self-reported somatic complaints, social anxiety, depression, and a tendency to worry or ruminate" (https://www.researchgate.net/publication/318919569_Your_Brain_Becomes_Graders_in_a_School-Based_Mindfulness_Intervention).

Within my own daughter's ADHD challenges and journey, mindfulness has significantly helped her to increase self-regulation and focus because it literally places her in a happy place of more positive emotions, gratitude, and optimism. She can now even notice when her mind begins to stray off topic; she's learned how to proactively re-direct herself back to the task at hand. I even catch her reminding her baby sister, age 2, to get back on track, if her sister starts asking random questions when we are doing a story circle time or playing a game.

The above study and my own descriptions match what neuroscientists around the world clearly confirm about mindfulness and its close correlation to focus and self-regulation. In the technical sense, brain structures and functions directly involved in self-control are positively modified or even re-wired with mindfulness training, especially in cases of mindful meditation. To illustrate, there is convincing evidence to verify the positive effects of MBIs in children as well as adults (https://www.ncbi.nlm.nih.gov/pubmed/29356899). More schools are integrating mindfulness into curricula and teachers are becoming trained and certified to utilize it in the classrooms at all levels nationally and globally. Acclaimed actress Goldie Hawn is one of the world's leading mindfulness proponents; she even cites how it not only helped her to parent her own kids and grandchildren with more confidence but also to overcome her personal and professional lifetime battles with mild dyslexia.

On the home front, how can you guide your kids toward greater focus and self-regulation today? While I am not a huge proponent of TV for kids, I must give a major shout out to the show called *Daniel Tiger's Neighborhood* for cleverly and effectively teaching self-regulation in such a fun, creative, engaging, and inclusive way. Using songs and multicultural characters, my daughters have learned such empowering lyrics, "When you feel so mad that you want to roar, take a deep breath and count to 4," and it works like a charm for those younger ones in your families! Remember how mindful Dorothy was despite the perils of her journey in *The Wizard of Oz?* You, too, can be that persevering against ADHD!

For older teens, distractions like having them walk the dog around the block, work on a puzzle or obstacle course as a family, take out the trash, run an errand to another teacher's room, or help address an envelope can also diffuse some anxious or aggressive emotions.

On the flip side, I uncovered some shocking and downright terrorizing studies that linked poor self-control in childhood to long-term, detrimental impacts. For instance, experts reported negative health, hindered academic achievements, and higher rates of criminality among preschoolers who struggled with self-regulation in their early lives. Disturbingly, these same kiddos were more likely to have substance dependence, financial troubles and a criminal record at age 32 (https://www.ncbi.nlm.nih.gov/pubmed/29356899). These studies are so menacing, so why not let mindfulness try to combat them?

Going back to our *Wizard of Oz* allusions, those claims are totally stuff from *the Wicked Witch of the West* that we don't want to happen to our sweet children, terrific tweens, or talented teens. After such a blast of bad news, how can we find hope and that cruise control of self-control?

Well, the good *Glinda* news is that focus and self-regulation can both be trained, thanks to mindfulness. Start by trying this simple technique and teach yourself and your kids this phrase and mantra, "I'm Not My Thoughts!" In turn, we can easily train and reprogram our monkey minds and befuddled brains.

Winston & Seif (2017) also posit in their book called *Overcoming Unwanted Intrusive Throughts: A CBT-Based Guide to Getting Over Frightening, Obsessive, or Disturbing Thoughts* how a mindfulness strategy can help tweens and teens get "unstuck" from out of control or irrational beliefs as we emphasize to our kids that they are "…just thoughts, and don't necessarily mean anything." Apply this cruise control concept this week and see if it makes a difference in focus and self-regulation. Save the glue for all those art projects, not our kids' brains!

Some additional tips include these strategies that I have devised into a *Mindfulness* acrostic poem to remember them more creatively:

M is for Meld the heart: When kids have ADHD, it is so easy to become trapped in the physical and mental manifestations. However, it is critical not to forget to employ a whole child concept because heart work is at the core of mindfulness. In turn, be *heart smart* as you meld the heart with the life lessons to generate more focus and self-regulation in kids, tweens, and teens.

Is for Initiate the pause button: Hitting pause is such a small but significant step to integrate more mindfulness for focus and self-regulation in kids with

ADHD. In Chadwick's (2019) article, "Miraculous Mindfulness With Kids: Accessing the Heart of the Matter," the author highlights the value of taking time daily for pauses to re-set the brain, activate focus, redirect concentration, and hone self-regulation.

As far as what this pause can look like, you might encourage kids to place a hand on their hearts. Smile. Breathe deeply into their bellies. At the same time, direct them to energetically breathe in and out through their hearts for a minimum of 30 seconds. It is just an easy exercise a few times a day to potentially increase mental stamina and better mind control overall. Think of it as a remote control's pause button for your parenting programming and patience!

N is for Nurture anologies. Mantras are a big part of mindfulness, but this jargon can sometimes intimidate kids at times. In my own experiences as a parent and educator, I like to make a simple one with kids, tweens, or teens collaboratively. Give them the sentence starter to show how they can autonomously and mindfully regulate their own minds with "My brain becomes a ____." Here are some examples that my teens formerly constructed: "My mind becomes a peaceful river." "My mind becomes a radiant rainbow." "My mind becomes a floating feather."

Remember as parents and teachers to revisit kids' analogies, post them, and refer to them often as teachable moments to build healthy habits in kids with ADHD holistically.

D is for Declare your intentions: The mere reference of a "goal" can often be boring to kids with ADHD, especially since they are often so bombarded with IEP goals and benchmarks at school. How does an intention work? Try asking them instead to declare their intentions, which is much more affirmative and accommodating.

In the (2017) book called Setting Your Intentions, Burdick & Honos-Webb (2017) identify how this skill is linked to better focus and overall success (p. v) with self-regulation aptitude. Start by having kids write down their intentions, discuss or state them, and/or then visually posting them for practice and retention.

F is for Find guided meditations: Find some audio examples or even online ones that will evoke focus and calm among kids, tweens, and teens with

ADHD. Some parents like to use a chime or bell to cultivate breathing and mini meditation sessions. My daughter's favorite is Amy Saltzman's *Still, Quiet Place* CD. Headphones or ear buds, anyone? Pandora also has some amazing music that is relaxing, free, and perfect for augmenting self-regulation.

To further validate this strategy with research, results from a (2009) British study also credited the immense, holistic benefits of meditation on students who have ADHD: students were calmer, less anxious, and had better memory skills after meditating twice a day for 10 minutes (Marley, 2009, p. 15), for example.

U is for Use a mindful symbol: My child has a rainbow pebble, for example, that she keeps in her backpacks and pockets sometimes when she's facing a challenging task like a timed test or experiencing trouble when sitting through a church service. This tangible, sensory symbol is small but big enough to remind her to focus in stillness like the pebble and allow others to see her vibrant colors. What will your kiddo's symbol be?

L is for Learn with games: One sensory game, in particular, can assist with focus and self-regulation in younger kids. It is called the Head-Toes-Knees-Shoulders (HTKS) and was developed to facilitate the behavioral aspects of self-regulation such as "controlling and directing actions, inhibitory control, paying attention, and remembering instructions for children ages 3½ to 6½ years" (Viglas & Perlman, 2018). It embodies 3 parts with the same instructions and scoring. The first part begins with two paired rules: "touch your head" and "touch your toes." The child is instructed to switch the rules by responding the opposite way. Two points are scored for following the instructions correctly (i.e., child touches one's toes when instructed to touch one's head).

How is it scored? 1 point is allocated for "self-correcting" (i.e., child makes any motion toward the incorrect response but then makes the correct response instead); 0 points are earned if the child touches the incorrect body part (i.e., either the child does not touch the correct body part at all or he/she touches the named part rather than the opposite one" (Viglas & Perlman, 2018). The main goal is to score at least 4 points to excel to the next round. Hey, it also teaches math, so it is a win-win on academic levels, right?

To simply it, I see it as basically a spinoff of "Simon Says" in the sense as the second part has the same instructions but with different paired rules like "touch your knees" and "touch your shoulders." It is also beneficial for practicing those listening and other affective skills like turn-taking and team work, too! Team works makes the dream work, right?

Games should be embraced, not merely discussed as child's play. In reality, research by Wegrzyn, Hearrington, Martin, & Randolph (2012) also supports brain games as a convincing nonpharmaceutical aternative for the treatment of ADHD, as discussed in the *Journal of Research on Technology in Education* (https://digitalcommons.kennesaw.edu/facpubs/2654/). Their (2012) study specifically required teen participants with ADHD to play "brain games" for a minimum of 20 minutes each morning before school for 5 weeks. Various tools like electroencephalograms, parent and teacher reports, researcher observations, and participant self-reports were used to assess the findings. In the end, the researchers asserted how the daily use of brain games can potentially help to strengthen teens' focusing ability and executive functioning with ADHD (https://digitalcommons.kennesaw.edu/facpubs/2654/). Game on, everyone!

N is for Never too late: Teach the notion that it is never too late to rewind or allow a mindful do-over. In kids with ADHD, they will likely not get it right the first time, so pausing and allowing them to fix, revise, and literally do over can really help with focus and self-regulation. It also tends to produce greater accountability and behavioral management. My daughter calls it her re-mix! Maybe she will be a future deejay?

E is for Engage in visualization: One mindfulness teacher describes how it helped her students to calm down easily and effectively re-set through visualization: "When I asked Aman if he saw a picture in his head when he concentrated on his breath and, if so, what it was, Aman answered "yes" and drew a stick figure sitting cross-legged on a cloud with a smile on his face. Aman showed an ability to concentrate in class and a precision in describing his feelings that did not appear in his writing, a skill that was difficult for him" (Bertolini, 2017). Mind over matter really does *matter* when it comes to ADHD, so paint, mold, and draw away! Zentangle, anybody?

S is for Sketch It: Drawing is another fabulous way to embed more focus and self-regulation into kids with ADHD. Bertoloni (2017) remarks how children's drawings serve as "a window into their inner lives, revealing their emotions, perceptions, and conceptions of the world." Pick up some supplies at the local dollar store and let your kids experiment with their emotions and mental concentration. Make Cyndi Lauper proud and show your "True Colors!"

S is for Selfie: Ditch the technology for a few minutes, but embrace the smiling concept. It is truly amazing how smiling will not only boost one's mood, but also uplift those around us, so try more smiling with your kiddos and see what follows. Say cheese!

Chapter 7: From Trippin to Road Tripping: Mindfulness for Stress Management

"Be happy in the moment, that's enough. Each moment is all we need, not more."

— *Mother Teresa*

After obtaining some easy and excellent ideas about how to use cruise control with your kids with ADHD from Chapter 6, let us now practice a bit more in this chapter to further extend your confidence. Are you frustrated, lost, angry, and despondent presently over your child's stress levels that never seem to level out? Is your tween or tween *trippin* over grades, body images, peer relationships, dating, clothing, allowance, curfews, and other issues? My oldest daughter with ADHD is constantly battling me when it is bath time and already becoming a mini fashionista like Tyra Banks or Heidi Klum as far as her daily clothing choices, so I am all about more mindful than manic parenting, mentoring, teaching, and coaching suggestions!

In sum, *let's stop trippin and start road tripping* down the *yellow brick road of resilience!* Try some of these simple techniques and browse the references on your own for culminating more stress management. Let us seek to chillax those ADHD conflicts and hot messes!

- **Quotable Quotes:** Just as Chapter 7's Mother Theresa quote motivates and diffuses my own stresses, ask your child, tween, or teen to keep post its with uplifting quotes, make copies of inspirational words, display or create mindful artwork, scrapbook together, or devise other visual reminders of motivational quotes or mantras to find one's center and peace against stress. Tell them that they can use technology to find them, and they will likely be more motivated to participate.

For older kiddos, I allowed them to make friendship bracelets and henna tattoos with empowering words, and they loved those ideas! When working with urban and at risk teens, we actually made group "graffiti walls" with inspirational quotes, and it was a memorable, successful activity for teens with ADHD.

- **Math Mania:** No, this tactic does not involve quizzes or math drills, but I learned this simple grounding technique at a teacher's workshop and use with often with my kiddos. It is called 5-4-3-2-1. Feel free to tweak if to suit your child's age and ability. You ask them to verbally or in writing recall 5- Things You Can See, 4- Things You Can Touch, 3- Things You Can Hear, 2- Things You Can Smell, and 1- Thing You Can Taste. It is not about the digits but about taking a moment to pause, decompress, and truly recognize one's surroundings in the now.

When tweens and teens with ADHS are running high on purely raw emotions or rage, plus hormones blended in the mix there, too, they often cannot think rationally. This very sensory-rooted exercise is great for giving them a reality and safety check.

- **Nurture in Nature:** Mother Nature is truly an underrated stress reliever and holistic healer, one that's totally cheaper than an expensive spa day, right? Various studies illustrate the immense benefits for better coping among kids, tweens, and teens with ADHD from merely interactions outside in nature. One (2008) study called "Spending Time With Nature Reduces ADHD Symptoms, Study Shows" from the *Annals of the American Psychotherapy Association* reveals how there is a possible close link between spending time in nature and reduced symptoms of ADHD. The study depicts how children with ADHD actually "exhibited better concentration and improved attention spans after taking a walk through a green environment" (p. 6). Do not merely wait for Earth Day to nurture yourself and your family in nature today!

Get creative and go old school on this one, folks. First of all, be kind to unwind, which means that you must flip off the TV and unplug all gadgets to truly nurture your family in nature. Take a walk, go for a hike, stroll, job, skate, or bike ride around the block or park. Pick some flowers, catch butterflies, find rocks, dig in the dirt, catch fireflies, throw around a Frisbee, play mini golf, swim, you name it! Depending on your area's climate, you can snowboard, ski, create murals with sidewalk chalk, collect rocks and catch butterflies or blow bubbles. Volleyball or badminton, anyone?

- **Zoo Crew**: Make deep breathing exercises a ritual. For the younger kiddos, modify it a bit to become more kid-friendly by allowing the wee ones to select a favorite toy or stuffed lovey. Research by Gale (2017) from the acclaimed *Harvard Business Review* finds that you can even have the younger kiddos place the item on their bellies as you guide them and verbally count how many times the animal (or toy) rides up and down to match their breathing (https://hbr.org/2017/11/how-busy-working-parents-can-make-time-for-mindfulness). If your house or life feels like a zoo due to ADHD, then switch gears with some deep breathing today. Experiment with this makeover into a *zoo crew*!

- **Bubble Guppies:** No, not the adorable cartoon version, but the old school fun and pastime. Manage stress in kids with ADHD with bubble solutions and some wands. Kids are often more apt to enter the mindful world with this type of breathing and literal exercise. Studies from the (2019) article called "Good, Calm Fun" in *Prevention* also reiterate that "If your child is having a tough day, ask her to notice how she is feeling: sad, worried, mad? Then encourage her to take a deep breath and blow all the icky feelings into the bubbles, letting them float away. Do this several more times, then talk about whether her feelings are starting to get better." Popping bubbles can *pop* away a ton of stress!

- **Ain't No Moutain High Enough:** In the same article mentioned above, parents can use bubbles with older kids who won't be tempted to suck in bubbles through a straw. Simply using a bowl, straws, and some organic dish soap, place roughly two tablespoons of dish soap into a bowl and add about 2-3 inches of water. Then have your child put his or her straw in the water and take a deep inhale through the nose. Challenge him or her to create the biggest bubble mountain to combat stress on the exhale. Research finds that this type of sensory strategy tend to help "boost her thoughtfulness and focus" (Good, Calm Fun, 2019) immensely. Plus, who doesn't really love bubbles?

For all the *American Idol and Voice* fans out there and Voice, you can also sing "Ain't No Mountain High Enough" if you are more musically inclined! Honor the version by Diana Ross or the original with Marvin Gaye! No lip-synching, ok?

- **Gumby Moments:** Add more stretch breaks and frequent walks to break the monotony, anxiety, or stress of a task. Be like Gumby and take a stretch break!

- **Having a Ball:** Stress balls usually work wonders when kids squeeze them as stress builds and accumulates. They are an easy, affordable, accessible, and mindful option. My daughters love Play Doh, clay, kinetic sand, and all the stretchy stuff out there on the market right now to calm and manipulate. Experiment with what works for your kiddos and *have a ball* in the process!

Chapter 8: School Days: Home Strategies for Academic and Vocational Success

The principle goal of education in the schools should be creating men and women who are capable of doing new things, not simply repeating what other generations have done; men and women who are creative, inventive and discoverers, who can be critical and verify, and not accept, everything they are offered."
— *Jean Piaget*

Coupled with Chapter 7's stress management tactics, I want to now overview some *school days'* survival tips and strategies for academic and vocational success in students with ADHD to try at home. As Piaget's quote embodies, we must encourage kids as lifelong, critical, and creative learners. These tips are necessary to introduce, integrate, and practice at home repeatedly.

Similarly, Hamilton & Astramovich (2016) specifically advocate in *Education* how kids with ADHD often seem to experience major "academic challenges and interpersonal difficulties which may impact their educational success" (https://eric.ed.gov/?id=EJ1104213). In my teaching tenure, I sadly saw many students wrongly dismissed as lazy or uncaring when in fact their ADHD hindered them from appearing like diligent students who were organized, punctual, and focused. For these reasons, this chapter is really essential to level the playing ground academically for your kids, tweens, and teens with ADHD first at home.

In addition to cognitive skills, parents should also revisit tactics from earlier and upcoming chapters that also integrate conflict resolution, communicative effectiveness, individualized homework assistance, etc.

In sum, here are some kid-friendly ideas to use and modify at home:

- **Calendar Guy/Gal:** Model for your kids and help them from an early age to use a planner, agenda, or calendar to track and record daily activities, homework chores, deadlines, etc. Calendar cool will keep you from feeling like a fool in school! Most schools have policies in place for how kids will track assignments and homework, so be sure you tag team with them for the best results. Remember the expression, "It takes a village?" Well, that sentiment is so true when working with kids with ADHD and other challenges!

- **Chunky Monkey:** While this title may look like a new ice cream flavor, it refers to the act of chunking or segmenting a task into smaller parts with frequent breaks. If a kids, tween, or teen with ADHD has an important research project, book report, experiment, or essay due, divide the task into manageable "chunks" with milestones. Be sure to celebrate as your child reaches each one.

I also recommend creating roadmaps for tasks with kids and asking essential questions such as "What do you have to do first?" I also like to use a white board with dry eraser markers to visually and tactilely demonstrate with kids collaboratively. This strategy helps to diffuse the monkey brain moments that stifle productivity and lead to procrastination.

- **Tick Tock:** Timers, reminders, and alarms might become your new BFFs for helping kids with academic and work tasks. Time management skills are so imperative, so start young with them. Tick tock, you don't stop reinforcing the value of time management. Which one/ones will you try this evening at home?
- **BFF: Buddy System:** Discuss the value of having a study partner or buddy, especially when kids are absent to get the missing work, review cooperatively for examples, peer edit essays, etc. Because kids, tweens, and teens struggle with social skills, do not rely upon them to be the ones to find the buddy. Ask the school to help and connect with reliable and positive peers but do it on the down low so it does not embarrass or draw attention to your kids, especially older ones.

I also recommend asking about Big Brother and Big Sister partnerships that your school may have with the community to assist with tutoring and mentoring.

- **Goalie:** Similar to road maps, as cited above to enhance kids' organization and time management, parents should also emphasize the need for goal setting at home, especially among older tweens and teens. Goals can drive or detonate our decision-making and can impact our actions. You do not need to be athletic or a soccer star to devise some effectively.

In brief, research praises goals for enabling the "stick-to-it-ness" that precede when a good habit is formed. McCarthy, Collins, Flaherty, & McCarthy (2017) in their article entitled, "Healthy Eating Habits: A Role for Goals, Identity, and Self Control," clearly suggest how changes are actually seen to occur medically "…at a neurological level with behavioral control moving from the goal-directed associative network to the context-directed sensorimotor network" (https://onlinelibrary.wiley.com/doi/abs/10.1002/mar.21021).   Thank God, there is no test on that part because that is a ton of medical jargon, right?

To simplify this vital suggestion, just remember to set your goals, state them, repeat them in writing, and also post them visually for increased retention in kids with ADHD.

- **Log It:** Since behavior is closely aligned to academic success, keep a behavior log to document any triggers, patterns, behaviors, interventions, strategies, and situations. It is easier for us as adults to react from emotional places to our kids, tweens, and tweens, so having facts and concrete evidence is so beneficial to ground us objectively. Where is your notebook? High tech parents can use phone notes, too. Make it work for you!

To reiterate a key feature to keep in mind when you are logging, try to always include the positives and efforts by kids. Do not merely list the negatives or outcomes.

On a collaborative and networking note, this log can further serve as a valuable tool when working with school, developing IEP goals with staff, and even discussing with medical professionals to sustain a team effort. Let us learn to log it with love!

- **Say My Name:** Make Destiny's Child proud and *say* all academic directions aloud; review vocabulary, and practice skills verbally to help kids with ADHD and task initiation. The use of verbal cues must accompany any written directions to jump start homework, studying, projects, test prep, etc.

I will admit that you can feel more like a parrot than a parent when using repeated directions with kids, tweens, and teens with ADHD, but stay centered, remained in the present, and be mindful during the process.

- **Cue Cards:** Use visual cues to prompt kids with ADHD to indicate start and stop assignment times, key vocabulary words, and so on. Here's your cue, folks!
- **Story Glory:** Read social stories to increase coping strategies. There are tons of great ones on Youtube.com or check with your local library. Which social story will be your kid's *story glory?* If your kid is more of a classical fan, then the old-school ones that we learned as kiddos are totally applicable still.
- **Metacognition:** This fancy term infers that one can think about thinking. It's a key part of helping kids with ADHD, so have your child explain how he or she solved a math problem or ask him or her if there's an alternative way to address a science project, English essay, health assignment, etc.
- **Chill Zone:** Designate a cool-down area in your home when academic battles or tensions happen. Have access to calming music, comfy textures, and so on.

You can also refer back to Chapter 7 for additional refreshers. You do not need for them to don fur or gloves to find a chill zone in your house or apartment!
Keep ear buds and/or headphones handy for all the auditory learners; use manipulatives such as Koosh balls or hand exercisers, as applicable. Let's chill!

Chillaxing is also rooted in research. For example, based on expert advice from Schipani (2008) in *Scholastic Parent and Child*, staying calm is paramount for any family member, parent, coach, mentor, teacher, or professional when working with kids with ADHD since "No one can think clearly when they're overwhelmed, and kids with ADHD are already having trouble accessing their thought processes. So when you further inflame them by yelling and engaging them in a light, nothing is accomplished. If you find yourselves in a meltdown situation, try to stay calm. Have everyone retreat and relax, and make an attempt to discuss it later, when everyone's calmer" (p. 68). Let's chill together and channel our inner Icelandic vibes!

- **Class Act:** As age appropriate and individually applicable, use behavioral contracts, positive reinforcements, incentives like sticker charts, and token reward systems to prioritize academic progress. Which ones do your kids prefer?

What is a token reward system? Also known as the token economy, Mautone, Lefler, & Power (2011) explicate in *Theory Into Practice* how it operates using the basic premise that tokens are frequently provided to the targeted child, contingent upon the occurrence of appropriate behavior. They can be exchanged at a later time for valued   reinforcers (https://www.researchgate.net/publication/51731976_Promoting_Fami If your kiddos love earning those tickets and tokens at amusement parks and arcades, then you might want to utilize this system at home. On a personal note, sticker charts work well with my preschooler, but earning extra time on the computer, a kid's choice day with family, time at the library, or another incentive might work better with older kids. Think outside the box!
A big part of the success of whichever system you choose is to constantly provide attention, positive feedback, and constant praise when your child with ADHD is on task and/or masters a skill successfully.

- **Stick It:** Add luggage tags to backpacks and book bags to remind students what to bring home to combat disorganization from ADHD. Focus on checklists and to-dos. Make Sugarland's "Stuck Like Glue" your parenting mantra for organization!

Again, Schipani (2008) further declares how organization is

indispensable for mindfully facilitating academic and vocational success in kids, tweens, and teens with ADHD: "I like to say that kids with ADHD need surrogate frontal lobes. That's your job, and the job of the school. The school can help your child organize his work while he's there, and make sure it's all in place for you, and then you can pick it up when he gets home. The key is that this isn't something you'll do once, but over and over again" (p. 68). Stay calm and model persistence.

- **Tap Dance:** While this suggestion does not mean enrolling your kiddo in actual dance classes, you can add sponges or mouse pads on desks for students who like to bounce, shake, or tap to allow them to channel physical motions when studying. Tap out any school tension or homework anxiety!
- **Rainbow Connection:** Invest in an array of colorful folders, labels, binders, and highlighters to enrich your child's organization. For my young girls who cannot read yet, I use picture mats and visual file folders. Let your colors shine on!

During my work as an educator, I have keenly discovered that many adults often try to do all the organizational legwork for the kids, tweens, and teens with ADHD, but it is equally essential to start young and get them actively involved in the process, too.

- **Class Act:** Roleplay and formulate scripts together to rehearse problem situations and how to advocate for oneself at school. You don't have to make your home a Broadway musical, but practice does make perfect. Look for social stories online, especially on Youtube.com and readers' theater scripts at your local library. If your child is a writer or super imagination, allow him or her to write some to perform puppet shows, monologues, etc. All the world's truly a stage! Get a glimpse of Shakespeare to promote those critical academic skills at home!

As mentioned recurrently within this book, kids, tweens, and teens with ADHD often struggle with adhering to deadlines, demonstrating punctuality, maintaining regular attendance, keeping focus, finishing projects, etc. For this reason, you can guide them academically and vocationally with some of these fantastic tips from this chapter.

To reiterate, Schipani (2008) openly acknowledges that coping with ADHD for all parties and family members is indeed a major journey as "It's not something that gets fixed overnight; it's not like dropping off a car at the mechanic's. One problem some parents have is that they are more than happy to help, but then they may think, "How will he ever learn if I keep organizing for him? If we keep him from sinking, how will he ever learn to swim?" But the fact is, "sink or swim" only works if you know how to swim. If you can't, you just sink. You're his safety net. And falling without a net is just too big a punishment" (p. 68). This book will better allow you to *win* and triumph using these resources, tips, and tools.

Chapter 9: Taking the Wheel: Mindfulness for Self-Esteem

"Confront the dark parts of yourself, and work to banish them with illumination and forgiveness. Your willingness to wrestle with your demons will cause your angels to sing."
— August Wilson

After learning about some academic success tips to try with your kiddos at home from Chapter 8, it is also vital to incorporate mindfulness for self-esteem. Let us now investigate some useful methods to help kids *take the wheel* and mindfully master positive self-esteem in Chapter 9. We presently live in such a wicked, weary world with so much bullying and cyberbullying and multiple mental health problems, such as eating disorders, self-harm, suicide, drug use and abuse, teenage sex, crime, etc. Therefore, we must take a mindful *detour* and disseminate how self-esteem is such a key part of development and holistic health for kids with ADHD.

Are you slightly concerned that this type of psychological work is out of your league as parents or a bit too clinical or touchy feely? Well, I assure you that self-esteem strategies are extremely necessary and of the utmost importance for all children to possess positively and proactively. You do not have to hold a doctoral degree or be a complete Dr. Freud to apply self-esteem tactics at home successfully.

Likewise, Moore (2010) maintains in *Academic Leadership* how kids with ADHD can greatly benefit from socioemotional perks related to mindfulness (p. 27). Without too much medical mumbo jumbo, because ADHD impacts brain regions that manage emotions properly, kids with ADHD often struggle with emotional intelligence, lower self-esteem, increased peer rejection, and other adverse effects. We need to directly find ways to bridge those brain gaps, which is what mindfulness essentially does by serving as what I like to think of as "the good glue" to bind it all together cohesively.

This glue metaphor that I have devised is actually close to what experts discuss as far as neuroscience. While I do not want to get too lab coat clinical here, technically speaking, Moore (2010) further elaborates how brain circuits formed from our emotional habits are actually "...sculpted during critical windows of opportunity in childhood and adolescence. And, we leave those experiences utterly to chance" (p. 27). Are you ready to equip kids with more authentic and increased self-esteem?

Like the lovely Lion character from *The Wizard of Oz* who lacked and desired courage, we must bravely wrap ourselves and our kids with lots of love, empathy, compassion, and forgiveness in order to offer them fortitude and positive self-esteem to survive and excel in life.

When a child has any type of diagnosis, many of us as parents and family members sometimes tend to coddle or overprotect the kid, but we must allow our children *to take the wheel* on this road to resilience and maturity. My younger child has OCD, anxiety, and Trichotillomania, the hair-pulling disorder, so it is a daily struggle for me to be mindful, not mad. With mindfulness, we can easily and effectively help kids to feel better about themselves, more peaceful and accepting of who they are when they see us in this mindful, accepting mindset as adults.

Check out some of these creative and research-based tactics for building self-esteem in kids with ADHD using mindfulness:

- **Talking the Talk**: Self-talk is a viable strategy that's deeply enveloped in mindfulness. Have your kiddos make a list of all their talents, assets, strengths, skills, and gifts. Cue them with "I've got _____." For example, my daughter likes to say, "I've got my art." I've got this." Aim for 5-10, depending on one's age and ability.

  Similarly, because of my child's fascination with unicorns and dragons, I also use this self-esteem builder with her quite often: "I soar with _____." She often answers 'kindness,' 'friendship,' 'silliness,' and other attributes that make her proud of who she is as an individual.

- **Freebird:** Do not make life all about gloom, doom, and fear, but do try to encourage kids with ADHD that life is a struggle and process for everyone. Many kids and teens with ADHD often succumb to self-fulfilling prophecies, cycles of learned helplessness, and victim mentalities. Have them accept that life is not always a fairytale or rainbow colored circus. Acceptance is a critical component of mindful training.

- **Roar and Soar:** Like the Lion from the movie who eventually receives his courage, give your kiddos the wings of self-esteem to soar. Guide them to identify and diffuse any destructive, debilitating beliefs.

Specifically, have them practice using I-statements like "I am talented, I am kind, I am funny, etc." When you allow them to overhear you bragging about their skills and strengths, they will also be more apt to embrace this optimistic, "freebird" mentality. Make Lynyrd Skyrnyrd proud by boosting up kids to feel confident and free, not shackled to a diagnosis.

On a musical note, we love to do car karaoke to Katy Perry's motivational song called "Roar!" Songs from *The Lion King* also work well, too, to foster self-esteem and musical memories with kids, tweens, and teens! Are you ready to make Simba proud?

- **Happy Place:** You may have heard of the instruction "to find your happy place," right? Well, encourage kids that they don't need a mall or group of BFFs to find immense self-esteem and serenity. Instead, ask your kiddo, tween, or teen to sit "crisscross applause" on a pillow on the floor or in a cozy chair with one's back straight. Guide him or her to let one's shoulders drop. Then lead him or her to take deep belly breaths and close one's eyes gently. We need to model and allow kids, tweens and teens that it is okay and actually a beneficial activity to sit alone in silence because we reside in a world of nonstop motions, images, messages, etc.

There are also a ton of apps if the child is older and more independent. The goal in this exercise is to clear any negative thoughts that enter one's mind and distract one. Just a 10-minute refresher can make an immense difference. It will probably feel weird to your children at first, but try to foster an open mind and remind him or her that even the celebrities and famous athletes do it! My young

girls both love foot soaks as a calming bedtime ritual, for example.
Just as Dorothy used positive thoughts in her famous, "There's no place like home" mantra, we also need to find ways to guide our kids with ADHD to think positively and clear their minds to focus on what they really want in life.

- **Dive into DIY:** DIY is dominating in conjunction with the surge in a *back to the basics* lifestyle. As a result, try to do some good old-fashioned arts and crafts and PLAY with your kiddo to combat the ADHD wiggles. Blocks, puzzles, board games, model airplanes and cars, STEM projects, science kits, scrapbooks, card games, charades, and Twister, are all fun and affordable ways to make kids feel more confident, creative, competent, and connected. To illustrate, various research studies suggest how concentration tremendously tends to surge during any form of art or DIY since it tends to change "your focus to something more manageable and, as a result, you experience less distress" (https://www.psychologytoday.com/us/articles/201609/what-s-the-deal-adult-coloring-books).

Because kids with ADHD need those hands-on, immersive, sensory-based activities, DIY is the Emerald City! What will be your family's DIY date night? When can you add a staycation into the mix for more family mindfulness and bonding? Smores, anyone?

- **1 Step At a Time:** One of my most enlightening quotes about ADHD is from Knowles (2010): "ADHD is not necessarily the inability to focus. It's the inability to not focus on everything. If the teacher was trying to teach a lesson and the two kids behind me were passing notes, and the kid next to me was tapping his pencil, I would be paying attention to each one of those things. Because I was paying attention to all of them, I couldn't fully understand what the teacher was saying" (https://www.naesp.org/sites/default/files/resources/2/Middle_Ma

For this reason, ask your kiddos to address a challenge one step at a time. Imagine climbing a ladder. What is the first step? Close your eyes, visualize yourself doing, it. Such a premeditative approach is not only mindful but super empowering!

ADHD Muse: So many mindfulness students excel from the individualized attention and personal coaching. Kids, tweens, and teens, too, need a muse who will be steadfast and supportive in their journeys. Knowles (2010) also asserts how they must have a support system who recognizes the disorder "and, despite that, believe in them and know they can be successful. Weiss and Hechtman followed youngsters with ADHD into adulthood. They concluded, "When the adults who had been hyperactive were asked what had helped them most to overcome their childhood difficulties, their most common reply was that someone (usually a parent or teacher) had believed in them" (https://www.naesp.org/sites/default/files/resources/2/Middle_Matters/ How can you best fulfill this muse role?

My daughters greatly benefit from the use of hands-on checklists and even the use of charts and progress jars to visually depict mastery or completion of one set or section of tasks at a time. Manipulate the manipulatives to make focus fun!

- **Can Can:** Of course I am not referring to the Parisian dance style, but the value of using an "I can" attitude and mindset with kids. Studies by Storeygard (2012) from *Exceptional Parent* strongly maintain how labels such as ADHD may exacerbate an adult's tendency "to talk about the child's behavior" (https://www.questia.com/magazine/1G1-303227460/my-child-can), rather than truly understand, articulate, applaud, and build upon the child's strengths and interests.

To employ the "Can Can" technique, jot down 5-10 strengths that your kids possess and brag about them. Then have them identify 5-10 "Can Can" strengths and goals.

If kids cannot write yet, integrate drawing or just discussing for this one.

- **Sasquatch Strategy:** I call this one being a Yeti because you take a negative statement like "I'm no good at history." You then have the kid with ADHD reframe it into a "Yeti" with I'm no good at history-yet!" Adding this "yet" tag boosts self-esteem, helps in goal setting, and gives Bigfoot fans something to "Bravo" about, right?

- **Holla for Happiness:** Kids, teens, and tweens with ADHD need to know that they are much more than a label or diagnosis in a chart. In order to apply this fun strategy, channel your inner Pharrell song, "Happy," and ask your kiddos to brainstorm 10 hobbies, strengths, skills, activities, or interests that make them happy. When they can see their merits, their sense of self-esteem will also elevate. "Don't worry, be happy!"
- **Soundtrack of Your Life:** When kids have ADHD, emotions tend to cause them to feel like they're cast members in a Cirque Du Soleil show. To keep self-esteem intact, have kids compile a list of 5-10 songs that bring them joy, humor, hope, and happiness as if the soundtrack for their lives. You can even make an actual playlist for road trips and those times when they literally need to hear the songs to augment mood and self-esteem. Rock on with your family!

In my daughters' cases, they both adore the entire *Trolls* soundtrack. I can use any song to instantly perk up their moods and self-esteem. Music can bond us and also build such strong memories, so find some songs today to empower your kiddos from the mind, heart, and soul!

- **You've Got Mail:** Older kids can embrace literary and also self-esteem at the same time as you encourage them to write a letter to themselves to celebrate a recent accomplishment, strength, completed school year, etc. It is a great exercise to use in both short and long term to identify areas of resilience. No stamps are required for this one!
- **Arts Smart:** Encourage your kid to keep a written, audio, or video journal/ portfolio. What about scrapbooking? Kids will be able to express themselves more and make vital connections to self-esteem when we encourage them to reflect on the "aha" moments in life.

Similar to sports, writing, painting, music, dance, and other forms of fine art are repeatedly linked to higher self-esteem. Studies further commend the mindful act of creating to foster creativity and self-esteem since it "implies that there is something inside of us that has value" (https://www.psychologytoday.com/us/articles/201609/what-s-the-deal-adult-coloring-books). Let's all dive into become arts smart!

Along the same lines, my preschool daughter loves animals, so she keeps a wildlife log of all the animals that she sees in our yard. She cannot write yet, so she draws the animals. When we look back on all her drawings, she is so proud of her budding naturalist skills; as a result, her self-esteem has also increased drastically from this fun, educational, and easy exercise. Let us all aim to become a big more *arts smart* and savvy overall as parents, teachers, coaches, mentors, and family members!

Chapter. 10. Balanced Banter: Mindfulness for Communication and Social Skills

"Anything that's human is mentionable, and anything that is mentionable can be more manageable. When we can talk about our feelings, they become less overwhelming, less upsetting, and less scary. The people we trust with that important talk can help us know that we are not alone."
— Fred Rogers

Based on some of the self-esteem suggestions from Chapter 9, you will now be better able to holistically hone your kiddos' social skills and communicative abilities even more in this concise section of Chapter 10. Communication, as Mr. Rogers expressed in the quote above, is so essential for building and sustaining trusting relationships. Yet how can we communicate positively and proactively when our kids often struggle to sit still or incessant repetition of requests than can be emotionally and physically draining on adults?

To address communicative challenges, mindfulness could bring some balancing banter to families struggling with ADHD on an ongoing basis. In fact, Mautone, Lefler, & Power (2011) justify in *Theory Into Practice* why social skills are so necessary, and the authors particularly hone what happens during the testy teen years: "While all kids, tweens, and especially teens can become highly defensive, irrational, and emotional, kids with ADHD seem to be more prone to these communicative challenges based on brain functioning. Although the symptoms of ADHD directly contribute to academic and peer relationship deficits, risk factors in the family environment indirectly contribute to their lack of preparedness to perform competently in school" (https://www.ncbi.nlm.nih.gov/pmc/articles/PMC3195402/). This advice means to me that if we start when kids are young to foster positive, mindful, collaborative, and empowering social skills and communicative rituals as a family, we can set the stage for amazing results into teen years and adulthood.

Besides, Knowles (2010) reminds us again how children, tweens, and teens with ADHD tend to have highly stressful and conflictive interactions with their parents, teachers, and authority figures which sometimes make it "difficult for them to establish and maintain strong parent–child attachments" (https://www.naesp.org/sites/default/files/resources/2/Middle_Matters/2009/M Schipani (2008) also adamantly repeats how positive parenting can often be even more impactful on kids, tweens, and teens with ADHD than medication since there some main communicative to-dos to apply when dealing with them: "First: Keep it positive. It's a rare child who, in response to negative attention, improves his behavior or performance. That's even more true of an ADHD kid. You need to keep it positive, constantly find something to praise, and try to avoid useless shouting or punishments, which don't work" (p. 68).

To further build upon these hypotheses and tips, this chapter is also vital since it encourages me to embrace that mindfulness exercises can potentially improve kids' cognitive, psychological, physical, socioemotional, and behavioral domains. I would also like to add spiritual and financial since communication can make or break in career and vocational settings. On a physical domain note, Oaklander (2015) also remarks in a Time.com article how mindfulness can produce a ton of benefits through physical movement: "It can combat stress, protect your heart, shorten migraines and possibly even extend life" (https://time.com/3682311/mindfulness-math/). Let us clear any bickering banter and aim for *balanced banter* in our holistic households!

For these reasons, add a few of these Fab 5 tips to teach kids more mindful communication and social skills within your families and households today:

1. **Diffuser:** Diffuse with empathy. I-statements are always essential for adult to express, as echoed formerly in Chapter 9 to stimulate kids' self-esteem growth. When your kiddo is crushed about not being able to go to an amusement park due to severe thunderstorms, try adding an extra dose of empathy. Roleplay a response like "Wow, I know it's such a bummer, but what are a few indoor backup choices that might be cool, too?"

How does this diffuser help? When kids know that you can relate to their emotions and validate them, they are more apt to calm down. Choices, too, diffuse heat moments. Think back to the last major conflict in your household. How could the diffuser technique worked to fan those flames or tame those tears and fears?
Empathy is a trust builder, and communicative is deeply based on trust. Try empathy in large doses when you communicate with your

kids and watch what normally happens in a more mindful, positive direction.

2. **Flower Power:** Are you tired of your kids with ADHD always complaining and feeling negative about school, friends, and life? Well, I borrowed this communicative and bonding technique called "Rose, Bud, and Thorn" from Race & Piquet (2015), as featured in *Camping Magazine* (https://www.acacamps.org/resource-library/articles/stress-camp-no-never-three-mindful-practices-create-kinder-happier-healthier-campers-counselors).

While I am not a camper or "glamper" by any stretch of the imagination, this technique transformed me from a grumpy cat parent to a happy camper because it helps to form a habit or ritual with kids about reflecting upon their days and experiences.

Try this easy debriefing exercise daily by asking kids to recall their "roses" first as something good that happened today, a new achievement, a proud moment, or any positive from the day. Perhaps she made a new friend? Maybe he received a college acceptance letter today?

Next, then have them name a "thorn" or a struggle, a challenge, or a problem that plagued them today. Maybe your daughter could not complete her science experiment during class time? Perhaps your son did not have anyone to sit with him during the after school baseball game and felt angry and isolated?

Lastly, encourage your kid to talk about the "buds." Like the buds on a flower, these "buds" signify the goals that they can informally set with you or the action plan and steps to promote future blossoming and growing! What are some ways that you can try to use flower power at home today?

On the other hand, if flowers are not your kids' cup of tea as far as age, personality, or preference, then you surely can adopt it to reflect dinosaurs, monster trucks, ballerinas, sports, or whatever they love!

3. **1 and Then Done:** This one is excellent for younger kiddos. My kids have major verbal and emotional meltdowns when it is time

to leave a fun place such as a birthday party or any excursion to the park. My *1 And Then Done* technique gives kids the choice to select one more activity before leaving. This choice allows kids to feel like they have some control over one's fate, despite the fact that parents retain control in the big scheme of things. My girls might choose to go down the slide once more or play in the sandbox for a few more minutes. I empathize with them how making choices can be tough, but I believe in them to build a foundation for future problem-solving.

In turn, I then set a quick timer or alarm on my phone to hold us all accountable. When the timer goes off, I also act disappointed with big doses of empathy, so they are less apt to argue with a "timer" than with me using this clever technique. It also affords them the illusion of control or power that they crave to pick one more item when the ultimate time management is still in adults' hands. The social skill and communicative part is activated when you have them repeat and chorally respond with the "1 and then done," too. It is also a superb listening tool. Try it this week!

4. **Oprah's On**: How many of you were avid fans of Oprah's former talk show or still avidly watch her interviews online today? Of course kids' demanding and redundant questions can sometimes drive you crazy, especially among the little ones, but psychologists firmly remind us to address the "whys" mindfully. Emulate the grace with which Oprah communicated with her guests during her talk show run and her signature style is truly mindful. Because mindfulness is all about nonjudgmental acceptance and empathy, those qualities denote why she is still such an inspiration to me and so many others worldwide.

What were some other key features of Oprah's approach that parenting with ADHD can also benefit from trying? Specifically, Chopra's (2008) wonderful article called "Conscious Parenting" in *Scholastic Parent and Child* discusses the value of answering kids "whys" to build better communicative and social skills, trust, and rapport. Chopra (2008) argues that these daily encounters tend to formulate the foundation "for our children's choices and values. And, if we take the time to explore how words make people feel good or bad, or how forgiveness allows us to love and to let go of hurt, we are providing our children with deep life lessons" (p. 62). My daughter with ADHD often operates purely from emotionally charged and fueled feelings, so discussions with empathy and nonjudgement tend to de-escalate her mood swings and channel her back into a logical mindset. Let us try to *own it like Oprah* as far as communicative and social mindfulness and swag!

5. **Get Real**: As adults, we must *get real* with kids, tweens, and teens with ADHD on a daily basis (and often on many "seconds" as a basis, right?). Since authenticity is a major ingredient in mindfulness, try to always operate from a genuine place. I know it is tough when a teen might be cursing at you, a toddler is hurling food or toys, or a tween is having a complete meltdown over a flat iron or football game.

To maintain a grounded sense of reality, Knowles (2010) in an article from *Education Digest* urges us to integrate these reality checkers continuously and mindfully when communicating with kids. How do we achieve this goal? Knowles (2010) includes some simple but profound tips that have been my blueprints as a teacher and parent: "Remind rather than ridicule. Be flexible. Everyone doesn't have to be doing everything the same way at the same time. Remember that no one is perfect. Be patient. Keep your sense of humor. Never, ever give   up" (https://www.naesp.org/sites/default/files/resources/2/Middle_Matters/ Which one do you really need to embrace first as your primary parenting cheer and sanity saver to support social and communicative skills in kids, tweens, or teens with ADHD? I think they are all great and go-to coping mechanisms that we can all utilize. Let us strive to *get real* together! Remember that we can literally re-wire our brains, so starting with these communicative techniques is a wonderful launching pad.

Chapter 11: Move and Groove: Physical Strategies for Mindfulness

"We see in order to move; we move in order to see."
— William Gibson

Upon acquiring new ideas for communicating proactively, collaboratively, respectfully, and positively in Chapter 10, let us now switch gears a bit and examine some holistic ways to add more physical movement to culminate mindfulness in kids with ADHD in Chapter 11. Are you ready to *move and groove on the yellow brick road* more naturally and confidently to your destination of resilience?

In particular, numerous studies presently exist to depict the close and positive relationships between movement and increased ADHD management from global research. You do not have to be an athlete, dancer, trainer, or gym guru in order to integrate some of the simple suggestions. According to a (2019) article from *IDEA Fitness Journal*, the author states how movement of any kind can greatly elevate our moods (https://www.ideafit.com/fitness-library/donrsquot-let-bad-moods-sabotage-you). What a simple way to blend that mind-body connection that is so vital for ADHD coping skills, right?

So many students with ADHD excel in sports, drama, dance, and other areas of physical activities. I have included some examples that work really well with my girls and also from my experiences as an educator. Kindly note that many other movement and physically-based examples are embedded into other chapters, too, since the whole premise of mindfulness is a holistic, integrated approach and lifestyle.

Try at least one of these ideas at home and see what happens:

- **Frozen:** Make Elsa and Anna proud by playing freeze dance and freeze tag with your kiddos. Not only are you promoting mindful movements, but you are also practicing active listening, something that kids with ADHD struggle to master. You can also incorporate old school classics like "Mother May I?" and "Simon Says" which are still quite effective, relevant, and fun. Just "Let It Go!"
- **Hippity Hop:** This one does not involve the Easter Bunny, but

we can teach kids about boundaries from a young age by having them draw boxes with sidewalk chalk to reinforce the value of staying in their own proximity bubbles. Then play a game of hopscotch or leapfrog with the chalky boxes. Hip hop, anyone? You can also use crayons and paper as an alternative and play a game of leap frog.

This "box" exercise has assisted my daughter with ADHD so much. She is not only highly impulsive but also extremely social. She always wants to hug people, even strangers, so the "stay in your bubble" strategy has been extremely effective at school, among family members, and within social settings.

- **Laughter Yoga:** Before you start chuckling, yes, this concept is a real activity and mindful movement approach. To illustrate, Bennett & Lengacher (2008) from a highly clinical article within *Evidence-Based Complementary and Alternative Medicine (ECAM)* summon how laughter therapy and laughter yoga can often help to manage moods, increase self-esteem, combat insomnia, and other overlapping implications from ADHD (https://www.ncbi.nlm.nih.gov/pmc/articles/PMC2249748/).
  While I have tried a class or two devoted to laughter yoga, I am more prone to unwind on my own with a comic sitcom, funny book, or comedic podcast. I also like to have a coffee date or happy hour with friends or family to LOL!

However, you want to giggle, snort, or cackle, use humor and laughter when parenting your kids with ADHD today. It is truly the best medicine, right?

- **Walking Labyrinth:** This one may sound a bit gothic, but it is actually holistic. Apply mindful walking in whatever form or pace suits you the most. It does not have to be formal, but you can experiment by making obstacle courses, treasure hunts, or labyrinths. Have them really focus on moving with intention and gratitude on casual hikes, strolls, etc. Walking it out is one of the easiest techniques when tensions are high.
- **Dance Fever:** Regardless of the musical genre, it is fun and

effective to allow kids to freely dance with you. Have family dance parties regularly to release stress and foster mindfulness. Disco balls are not required, though!
- **ABCs of Movement:** Enlist your child's help and make a comprehensive list from A to Z of creative ideas to add more movement to your family's lives.

Here are my daughters' recent favorites: A is for aerobics, B is for Bowling, C is for Corn Hole, D is for Dodgeball, E is Elevator (My daughters, as mentioned, are ages 4 and 2, so they taught me this make believe game!), F is for Frisbee, G is for Golf, H is for Hula Hoop, and I is for Ice Cream Truck (Again, they are ages 4 and 2). Are you ready to make your ABCs with your kids, tweens, and teens to cope more calmly with ADHD?

Chapter 12: Peaceful Parenting: Mindfulness Tactics for Parental Stress Management

"There is no magic cure, no making it all go away forever. There are only small steps upward; an easier day, an unexpected laugh, a mirror that doesn't matter anymore."

— Laurie Halse Anderson, Wintergirls

Now that you are utterly energized from all the mindful movement and physical ideas from Chapter 11, Chapter 12 will present some peaceful parenting tactics for you as the adults to employ more self-care and holistic health to your lives and roles. When working with or parenting a child, tween, or teen with any diagnosis, especially ADHD, we often undergo real feelings of immense pressures, marital strife, physical and mental health struggles, time and financial management, guilt, anger, sadness, loss, frustrations, stress, blame, and other adult challenges.

As mentioned, mindfulness is not a magical cure or pill to swallow, but it can certainly melt away stress and anxiety, like *the Wicked Witch of the West* was dissolved by the water in the movie. Once you master the basics and accrue practice over time, you will see the results in yourself and your kids! Experiment today with at least one of these *Grateful 8 Strategies*. They are not listed in any particular order of importance, so feel free to mix and match:

1. **Under the Sea:** Whether you are a wondrous water baby or a lovely landlubber parent, it is so necessary to deeply and truly connect with your inner parental mermaid/merman and maintain a parenting model that is not all about perfection.

Keep yourself afloat and your head above the waters. Recognize that like water freely flowing, parenting a child with ADHD is not stagnant and/or a perpetually picture perfect or pretty pond.
Ride and let the waves and whirlpool of colorful emotions and evolving learning experiences exhilarate you and unveil your inner strengths amid the serious struggles (and sharks!). Do not forget to play and *splish splash* along with the way because humor will be your

life vest as you surf steadily in life, teaching, coaching, and parenting!

2. **Love Lingo:** This technique is also imperative. Use your words mindfully and compassionately. Do not fight fire with fire; do not allow words become weapons when parenting kids, tweens, and teens with ADHD. Of course this does not mean that you must speak in eloquent poetry and poise all the time, but learn love lingo.

Why? It can tenderly tame your tongue when we use love lingo instead. Following suggestions from Conscious Parenting experts, I have learned to take a moment literally since we as parents must really try and discern the difference between reacting to kids with ADHD from the centered state of who they are and from our own proud, parental egotistical worlds.

While this advice might sound a bit harsh, love lingo roots us in reality and empathy, so it affirms that we as adults have already had our own time to grow up and learn the ropes of this world. Thus, love lingo is powerful because it reminds us not to make it all about us as the adults. What does this mean? It does not encourage you to be a pushover or door mat, but try to not take everything so personally, although I know it is much easier said than done.

It also forces us to stop comparing ourselves to other parents, the Kardashians, and everyone else out there. Who cares what others think about us as parents and people? Be authentic and live in love in your own skin! You are not in a pageant or parenting competition, so learn love lingo for confidence and empowerment.

One way to employ better love lingo is to have some handy dandy one-liners when tensions are high to diffuse your own adult egos. My favorite one, for example, is "I love you too much to argue." It works like a charm with my kids, spouse, and family members. What will be your love lingo line/lines be? Think creatively and practice, practice, practice. Live the love lingo when you are "Livin La Vida Loco!"

3. **Pregnant Pause:** No, this strategy is not advocating a plan to conceive another bun in the oven, foster an entire football team, or adopt triplets, but I assure you that it is one of the easiest ways

to integrate mindfulness into your daily life routines and parenting approaches. Simply add a *pregnant pause* and breathe deeply when you feel overwhelmed, frazzled, angry, or ready to give up. Newport's (2018) article in *The Magazine For Addiction Professionals* offers an idea from the legendary guru, Thich Nhat Hanh, who advises us to stop and truly take a moment to envision or recite this mantra, "Breathing in I calm my body, breathing out I smile" (https://www.counselormagazine.com/en/columns/2018/columns/ dec-2018).

I love this idea so much that I actually suggest repeating it based on your age (or your kiddo's ages): so if you're 40, do it forty times! Words are so powerful, so "word up" with this holistic wisdom to cope with ADHD!

4. **Slow Your Roll:** Of course you can order some yummy sushi when you are overly stressed and over the parental edge, but this mindful strategy is equally imperative. Reduce and slow your pace as a family and parent. In general, Race & Piquet (2015) assert how our kids today are sadly growing up "in a culture that constantly stimulates the stress response — fight, flight, or freeze" (https://www.acacamps.org/resource-library/articles/stress-camp-no-never-three-mindful-practices-create-kinder-happier-healthier-campers-counselors). Take a moment tonight and look at your calendars objectively.

   Kids with ADHD can become overwhelmed so easily and over-stimulated. Don't let tons of back to back, crammed scheduled events, technologies, or rushing around everyday exacerbate the ADHD triggers. In turn, *slow your roll*, ya'll! Take a minute and critically reflect upon this week's calendar. Talk to your kiddos about which ones to prioritize. Discuss together ones to possibly modify or delete in order to spend more face time with your kiddos, not Facetime, the app. Slow your roll before stress takes a toll!

5. **Balancing Act:** Parenting in a mindful manner does not mean being a cop or being a lenient buddy to kids 24/7. In actuality, it

is truly about respectfully setting limits and reinforcing your authority with "I'm the adult here" (Southgate, 2002, p. 210). It does not always feel this way when parenting, so this helpful tip is one of my favorite pieces of advice for adults.

Similarly, the article, "Wonder Years," from *Essence* helps us to also realize that as early as 9 months, we must model and reinforce to children consistently which behaviors are acceptable and those that are not. If we are constantly frazzled and depressed when dealing with a kid's diagnosis, then we automatically model the negativity and toxic vibes that follow.
Think like a gymnast and find that proper balance; center yourself holistically and mindfully as a parent to keep your stress minimized and your confidence flying high amid ADHD!

6. **Chillax:** Taking a timeout is not just for kids. In reality, adults equitably need to take breaks in order to remain grounded and sane when parenting, coaching, mentoring, or treating kids with ADHD in any capacity or role. If your child is having a major meltdown, tantrum, diva session, or rebel without a cause chaos moment, I suggest using this technique on yourself called "Stop, breathe, and chill" as Francis (2008) advises in "Peaceful Parenting" from *Scholastic Parent and Child.*

When attempting to take my daughters today to lunch at Panera Bread, I sat with them on a small couch in the middle of a crowded mall while I was trying to order online, so we could skip the line and go straight to our table. I asked them to play calmly with their sticker books together while I ordered. In less than 30 seconds, a circus ensued: they rambunctiously used the public couch as a trampoline, started pulling each other's hair, kicking, pinching, and sobbing loudly. I then had to apply this technique to literally calm myself first before attending to their mall mania. When do you need to chillax the most as a parent? What are you currently doing to destress less?
 Along the same lines, this super strategy is heralded by many other psychological and educational experts. Again, Francis (2008) contended that, "Once you've reached a place of acceptance, add

some positive self-talk to swap "I'm going to snap!" with "I've got this" (p. 10)! Ready to chillax? What will be your self-talk phrases? Write them down now and start practicing, please.

7. **Bookworm:** Do not stop learning as an adult. Learn from resources, books, other parents and experts, etc. Arrange playdates with other families to share ideas. Find parenting books at your local library, on Kindle, or listen to a mindful podcast or webinar about positive parenting. Bookworm it, baby! Some of my most enlightening parenting tips come from parenting blogs because the writers are enveloped in the trenches daily.

8. **Pump It Up:** Exercise is so essential and something that parents need to maintain mindfulness, health, and sanity. I know many experts recommend striving for roughly 10,000 steps per day, but my personal goal is 7500. If you lack the time or funds to join a public exercise class or facility, I keep love the convenience and effectiveness of these online ones that I can do while my kiddos nap at https://www.fitnessblender.com/.

I swear, I am not receiving any promotional or monetary compensation for suggesting them. They have literally toned and changed my life and mental health. They are also free and readily adaptable to suit any level or need. *Pump it up* for parental patience and power in whatever way suits your style and preference.

Chapter 13: Toolbox: Methods to Try at Home for Mindful Kids, Tweens, and Teens

"The function of mindfulness is, first, to recognize the suffering and then to take care of the suffering. The work of mindfulness is first to recognize the suffering and second to embrace it. A mother taking care of a crying baby naturally will take the child into her arms without suppressing, judging it, or ignoring the crying. Mindfulness is like that mother, recognizing and embracing suffering without judgement.
— Thích Nhất Hạnh, *No Mud, No Lotus: The Art of Transforming Suffering*

Using the knowledge and ideas from Chapter 12 to keep parental stress in check, you can freely add more mindfulness tools to your toolbox. I love the idea presented in the quote above that we cannot possibly have a lovely lotus without also having the mud. This metaphor for parenting is something that I try to keep in mind, even on my darkest days. I also want to pass on this advice to you and build support.

In turn, I challenge you to try at least one of the following techniques this week from Chapter 13 since these tactics tend to merge theories and suggestions from all former chapters collectively. This chapter is short because all of the other practical ones give more elaboration and mindfulness methods.

- **The Nose Knows**: Calm your kids and selves with therapeutic essential oils. Aromatherapy is great, relaxing, and highly therapeutic, so try some holy basil, spearmint, lavender, etc. In reference to a Thai study, Huffington (2016) found that stress reduction was expedited after smelling lavender and literally "... slowing down our heart rate, decreasing our blood pressure and lowering skin temperature" (http://time.com/4269916/arianna-huffington-better-nights-sleep/). Home spa day?

- **Calm Boxes:** Younger kids, in particular, can benefit from making a calm box. My daughter's actual box is a bag that contains her favorite stress ball, a stuffed animal, her headphones, and other items that instantly release her stress. Kids who are artistic can draw, mold, paint, decorate, and/or build their own!

- **Oxygen Mask:** Add deep breathing exercises, mini meditations, body scans, and child yoga poses to the mix. Kids can start within finger breathing, where you line up each fingertip with the corresponding fingertips of the opposing hand. Direct them then to draw their fingers close together: and with the inhalation, guide them to expand their fingers, stretch them out, and aim to keep the tips connected.

On the exhalation, encourage them to let the fingers draw back together as the fingers follow the breathing in and out, as borrowed from Race and Piquet (2015) (https://www.acacamps.org/resource-library/articles/stress-camp-no-never-three-mindful-practices-create-kinder-happier-healthier-campers-counselors). Great oxygen mini masks and mittens for mindfulness, eh?

Chapter 14: Mood Foods: Holistic Eating for Managing ADHD

"One cannot think well, love well, sleep well, if one has not dined well."
— *Virginia Woolf, A Room of One's Own*

Similar to the sentiment expressed in Woolf's quote, mindfulness also targets this notion of mindful eating as a link to better holistic health. Once you have tried some of the home strategies from Chapter 13 and earlier sections, I bet you have now worked up an appetite, right? Forge the greasy fries and heart attack shakes; opt instead for some *mood foods*!

Recent studies by Yunus (2019) from the renowned *Exceptional Parent* have asserted how there is a possible link between ADHD and high sugar, salt, and fat intake when kids receive diets with only minimal whole grains, fruits and vegetables intakes (p. 24). Many findings specifically herald the benefits of a whole food plant-based (WFPB) diet with minimal or no processing for protection against ADHD, cancers, heart disease, osteoporosis, and other chronic conditions (Yunus, 2019, p. 24) as well.

While I am not suggesting a rigid *Biggest Loser* style diet or any particular dietary model, I want to offer some general *mood foods* and natural drinks that in this chapter that not only taste great but are healthier options for you and your kiddos as far as mindful eating. I also want to arm you with research and resources, so you can explore and take it to the next level as far as what is best for your particular family's needs.

Are you ready for some yummy suggestions? Let us find those aprons, ok?

- **Snack Attacks:** Make snack attacks healthy with fresh fruits and veggies. Make healthy smoothies together and add some chia and flax seeds to balance moods. *Masterchef Junior*, anyone?
- **Mr. and Ms. Clean:** This advice does not mean operating a pristine household free of dust bunnies and flawlessness, but it is about eating as clean as possible to avoid unnecessary additives and food colorings. Of course kids are attracted to the colorful, marshmallow, vibrant products that are often so full of crap. Yunus (2019) also divulges how we have a clear responsibility as

parents and the ones who typically purchase the food products to ensure that nutrition is clean for children, tweens, and teens with ADHD since "This is a controversial subject and, because we often have an emotional attachment to food, we are reluctant to look at this as an adjunct treatment" (p. 25).

Of course you can still serve an Oreo or ice cream to your family once in a while, but Yunus (2019) and other dietary experts warn how it is definitely likely that artificial food colorings play a major role in "the development of symptoms in some with ADHD. Some children with ADHD may also be sensitive to foods such as milk, chocolate, eggs, soy, wheat, corn and legumes, along with salicylate-containing foods such as grapes, tomatoes and oranges" (p. 25). For this reason, try to eat like Mr. and Ms. Clean as best as you can. Also keep a food log to document.

- **Diggity D:** There is "No Diggity" about it that Vitamin D is the superior sunlight vitamin that most kids, tweens, and teens often lack from excessive indoor gadget time, nutritional voids, etc. As a result, Laliberte's (2010) "Problem Solved: Winter Blues" from *Prevention* insists that we must all ensure that our family members are *digging it* with vitamin D proactively since it is closely linked to keeping our serotonin levels elevated and balanced (p. 48). This connection is something that is super important in kids, tweens, and teens with ADHD for critical brain balance and overall wellness.

Are you excited to dig it with D? Take a family hike, jog, stroll, or skate around the block. Find a local park and dive into the D!

- **Straight from the Hive:** Try warm milk with Manuka honey for a natural relaxer before bedtime with your kiddos. My girls really love it on bananas with peanut butter and chia seeds, too. You can also add it to evening herbal teas to evoke some sweet dreams and deeper sleep.

As a slight disclaimer, because of honey's sugary contents, be sure to just use a small amount, roughly the size of a poker chip. Just do not try to karaoke Lady Gaga's "Poker Face" song, or you might lose face with older kids! BEE holistic, BEE well, and BEE wonderful when you *try honey with your honey!*

- **Sugar High:** As adults, we really need to embrace the "You are what you eat" mindset with all kids, but specially those who have ADHD. In turn, closely monitor sugar intake with their candies, sodas, caffeinated beverages, and all those ooey gooey treats and desserts. Carefully monitor the amount of fast foods that you are serving to your families, not matter how tempting or timesaving it may seem. Studies encourage us to eat "clean" as clean as possible as opposed to relying on the fatty, greasy, overprocessed foods. Clean eating will naturally "eliminate unnecessary food additives such as artificial colors, flavors, sweeteners, and preservatives that do not add nutritional value and may contribute to ADHD symptoms. Limit sugar intake to 10% of total calories daily (roughly 6 teaspoons for children aged 2 to 19 years)" (Rucklidge, Taylor, & Johnstone, 2018, p. 16).

My own daughters recently attended a birthday party with tons of sugary cakes, candies, and fruity drinks. They then began bitterly bickering in the car on the ride home to no avail from all the junk in the trunk (literally). Are you eager to crush that sugary rush and move toward mindful eating? I have been baking and cooking with dates as a natural sugar alternative when I make muffins and other goodies lately. While I am not a professional cook or baker by any means, I encourage you to freely consult cookbooks at the local library or online that focus on mindful and natural ingredients to curb those sugar high sensations that tend to exacerbate ADHD! Be mindful when dining out and always look for healthier family options.

Putting a freeze on fast food addictions can be so instrumental. La Valle's (1998) pioneering article from *Drug Store News* also indicates how high sugar intakes can cause low blood sugar and chromium depletion. The fast food frenzy is really taking a toll on our kids as "The average American now consumes an average of 152.5 pounds of sugar in a year. That large soft drink at the drive-through window contains roughly 22 to 27 teaspoonfuls of sugar. It is reported that increased sugar intake actually increases urinary chromium excretion. Over time, this could have an impact on behavior" (CP13).

- **MOOve Over:** Dairy overload can often cause major digestive issues. When kids are literally plugged up, they can act out even more. To counter these tummy troubles, consider some new dairy alternatives like almond, soy, coconut, cashew, and oat milk. I also suggest adding probiotics to your kiddos' diets with more kefir, Greek yogurt, and other mood foods. In my daughters' cases, they have been extremely helpful to tame tummies and boost moods. Let us MOOve over mindfully!
- **Veg Heads**: You can opt for a Meatless Monday approach for more mindful family eating. Try to replace traditional noodles with veggies such as asparagus, zucchini, carrots, etc. Indulge in Brussel sprouts, cauliflower pizza crust, corns, asparagus, etc. Be a vicious veg head and also add more veggies to morning egg dishes, especially omelets.

Make the Jolly Green Giant proud and be a veg head of household more often to facilitate holistic health and happiness in all kids, but especially ones with ADHD! My oldest daughter adores making and eating kale chips with me. She has also recently been trying the freeze dried snap peas, too. We never know what they will like until we experiment, right? Go beyond broccoli and green beans on your next grocery run!

- **B Well:** Yunus (2019) again shows the correlation between inadequate vitamin and mineral intakes in ADHD, particularly with "Iron, copper, zinc, magnesium and calcium deficiencies are common in those with ADHD and itis theorized that this may affect the central nervous system. Nutrient poor meals and snacks are implicated as contributory for those with ADHD" (p. 25). What can you do to stop this vitamin and mineral void in your families?

In essence, it is also highly advantageous to ensure that your kids, tweens, and teens are getting enough B vitamins in their diets: B1 is linked closely to many key functions like immunity, heart support, and mental processing; B2 offers energy, hair, skin, and eye health; B 3 stabilizes our memories, moods, and hearts; B5 can keep cholesterol levels in check; B6 is a sleep reliever. Are you ready for some "Sweet Dreams" by Queen Bey?

Finally, buzz with B-12 for increased mood and energy management. My young kids love the "classic ants on a log" snack with peanut butter, cashew butter, sunflower seed butter, or almond butter slathered onto celery with raisins, dried cherries, or cranberries. Have fun in the kitchen and make Rachael Ray proud in a healthy and mindful way today!

- **Beanie:** While I am not talking about the cool, fashionable hats, try to eat more mindfully against ADHD with beans and legumes. Make black beans burritos, hummus with chick-peas, serve up some edamame, and add lentils or sunflower seeds to beam up your families' diets!

- **Magnesium Magnets:** Strive to add more magnesium into your family's overall dietary routines, especially in cases of ADHD. Studies describe how the average American is often highly deficient in magnesium "by about 70 mg daily. Magnesium is the calming mineral, since it is the principal mineral used to control the parasympathetic nervous system. There is also the potential for calcium deficiency. Many children complain of aching legs and will see positive results with the initiation of a well formulated multiple mineral supplement" (La Valle, 1998, CP13.). Get your *magnesium magnets* via food or supplements today!

- **Finding Nemo:** Set a goal to serve a fatty fish to amp up those Omegas and vitamin D 2-3 times a week. Yunus (2019) reminds us of compelling research that depicts how those with ADHD may also have "lower levels of omega-3 fatty acids and higher levels of omega-6 that may lead to inflammation and oxidative stress" (p. 25).

Accordingly, Evidence by Rucklidge, Taylor, & Johnstone, (2018) also suggests that supplementation with omega-3s and/or a broad spectrum of micronutrients (for those not taking medication) may be beneficial for ADHD symptom reduction, but it is so important that all "Patients should consult with their primary care provider before starting any supplement and with a dietician before changing their diet" (p. 15). Get your rod and reel in some *fishing* action in during family meals and snacks for more mindful eating.

In fact, salmon nuggets and fish sticks are always major hits with my girls! They also enjoy coconut shrimp with fun and tasty dipping sauces. How can you get your Nemo and Dory on and blast more fish in your weekly menus?

- **See for Yourself:** Fruits like pineapples, grapefruits, tomatoes, berries, mangoes, oranges, and kiwis, are a definite self-care saver for the blasts of vitamin C. I also recently discovered passion fruit, a rich source of beta-carotene and vitamin C, as recommended by the recent article aptly called "Mood Food" (2019) from *Daily Mail*.

My girls love to toss some seeds onto their morning yogurt parfaits. Try some today and *see for yourself* if your kids will likely say "Yay!"

- **Zing with Zinc:** Assist your kids with ADHD in the culinary department to better *zing* against mood swings, common colds, flus, and other physical problems. Simply add more fruits and vegetables rich in zinc to their diets daily.

Honor the great pumpkin! Don't wait for Halloween and toss some pumpkin seeds to kids' sandwiches, baked goods, cereals, oatmeal, yogurts, pastas, salads, etc. Experts praise them for reducing feelings of anxiety (Mood Food, 2018), something that kids, tweens, and teens with ADHD know all too well, right? Let's *zing* and sing with zinc!

- **Grain Brains:** Apply more whole grains to your family's meals regularly. Go for wheat breads, overnight oats, brown rice and pastas, quinoa, barely, granola, etc. Gravitate toward making some *grain brain* nutritional gains!
- **Happy and Hydrated:** I know you have probably heard this one a zillion times, but it is vital to reiterate the value of ensuring that

kids get enough water daily. If your kids will not drink water plain, have fun adding cucumber slices, lime, lemon, berries, mint, or other fun and tasty additions. Let us *hoot for hydration* happily and holistically!

Chapter 15: Destination Resilience: Mindfulness for Resilient Families

"The human capacity for burden is like bamboo- far more flexible than you'd ever believe at first glance."

— Jodi Picoult, *My Sister's Keeper*

Since you can now approach family meals, snacks, and lifestyle changes more mindfully and holistically using ideas from Chapter 14, let us pull it all together and approach the *Emerald City of resilience* against ADHD in Chapter 15. Whether you are in Kansas, Katy, Kauai, Kuala Lumpur, Kodiak, Kent, or Kyoto, we need more resilient families to empower our kids' lives.

For starters, families can definitely build and maintain resilience in a variety of mindful ways. I want take a quick detour on this parenting road trip and acquire more insights about what resilience is, why it's so essential for kids with ADHD, and various tips to build it. As the quote above embodies, we must use the bamboo metaphor to survive and thrive against the pressures of ADHD.

First off, what is resilience? To give you a helpful hint, you are already tapping into your own resilience as parents because you have purchased this book, so I am truly proud of you! I personally define resilience as the Gumby or rubber band quality that allows us all to bounce back after challenges, traumas, misunderstandings, failures, self-doubts, and conflicts.

To provide a more scholarly definition, Dillen's (2012) article from The *International Journal of Children's Spirituality* specifically cites resilience as the ability to bounce back in times of adversity and to react positively when faced with setbacks. What metaphor can you presently use with your child to demonstrate the necessary grit and tenacity to bounce back in life? I literally take an item as a manipulative and use it as a visual with kids. As a teacher and parent, I have demonstrated with a beach ball, scrunchy hair band, yoyo, and array of other props to reinforce this premise of resilience. What will be your power prop to *give props* to resilience?

Next, now that I have briefly defined what resilience is, I want to explore why it is so critical to boost this ability in kids, tweens, and teens with ADHD. As this book has repeatedly mentioned in former chapters, kids with ADHD face an entourage of physical, cognitive, psychological, socioemotional, spiritual, and behavioral challenges that warrant them to be flexible, adaptive, strong, and perseverant. It is almost as if a camera is on them 24/7 and a perpetual parade of paparazzi is hounding kids with ADHD, right? If you are a *Big Brother* fan, then you know that stressful vibe, right?

Likewise, Ginsburg (2011) in the book, *Building Resilience in Children and Teens: Giving Kids Roots and Wings*, even directly explains and proposes that resilience is the fourth "R" following the other essentials of "Reading, "'Riting," and "'Rith-metic" that kids must master today for lifelong learning and success in school, work, and life. This addition of resilience makes mindfulness an even more applicable skill to instill and practice at home starting from a young age.

To further convey the idea of resilience in my own household with a toddler and preschooler, I hopped on the popularity bandwagon of the unicorn trend recently. Specifically, when my daughter with ADHD becomes frustrated by failures or trapped into pits of perfectionism, I cleverly redirect her to consider her special "horn of magic" as a secret symbol; this allusion creatively and calmly reminds her of the radiant rays of resilience that deeply reside within her. It is such a fun and effective way to fan those flames of anger, chaos, and self-doubt.

When ADHD becomes challenging or overwhelming in your household next, what can you use as a symbol or shield to assist your child to summon the strength of resilience? When ADHD is a major barrier in school, social settings, home life, or work, establish a secret code or password to impart lessons of resilience. Sure, it is a bit silly but quite fun, trust building, and rife with resilience!

Finally, I will deliver even more ideas in this section, so feel free to check out this *Zen 10 list* of resiliency rockers to try at home with your kiddos, tweens, and teens. The suggestions are not listed in any particular order of importance, so feel free to mix and match:

1. **Mirror, Mirror:** While this tip is not only limited to fairytales, try to use books, movies, videos, and other pieces to teach, build,

analyze, and practice empathy with kids, tweens, and teens with ADHD. Allow kids to walk in another character's shoes to mirror feelings in others, discuss and accept others' experiences, demonstrate compassion, tolerance, etc. My daughters are much more excited to address empathy and practice when we talk about Elsa, Moana, Trolls, Smurfs, you name it!

Are you ready to get your book buzz on as a family? Movie night is the perfect time to cultivate empathy. Pop that popcorn, find your snuggly blankets, and forge a path to build empathy!

2. **Chores Galore:** Give kids, tweens, and teens daily chores and responsibilities to increase accountability and boost autonomy. Chores increase resilience because students see and experience how hard work pays off, despite the challenges. My daughters are already become skilled at folding laundry, setting and clearing the table, giving water to our kitties, etc. Chores help to increase character as well as alleviate boredom, a frequent claim among kids with ADHD!

3. **Brain Drain:** Calmly, collaboratively, and honestly talk and walk through problem solving aloud with your child. In fact, the brain drain technique is my own take on the value of brainstorming alternative resolutions in a mindful manner.

When my daughter was unfortunately being bullied at her school, for example, we completed a few brain drains together at home to create a concrete plan on what she could do to address it the next time it happened. I strongly advise you not to do all the work for the kids. The critical piece of this technique involves getting the kids to use critical thinking skills.

As far as my daughter's brain drain results, this technique not only helped to her express difficult emotions, but it also validated her feelings of alienation and shame. I also shared examples from my own life about when I was also bullied in school. She was then also able to clearly state and goal set by herself that her game plan for a future encounter with the mean girls and guys on the playground. In her case at age 4, she chose and vocalized these 3 options on her own: a. She could play alone on another piece of equipment. B. She could tell a teacher or aide. c. She could firmly say "no thank you" to the bullies. D. She could walk away and think, "I've got this" in her mind.

As a result of the brain drain, I was so impressed (and frankly a bit speechless) that a preschooler could actually exhibit such advanced resilience when it took me as an adult about 20 years to gain resiliency skills.

Moreover, we can smoothly guide kids to bounce back more effectively and independently if and when they can solve their own problems, rather than always allow adults to constantly coddle or fight fires for them. Remember you are a parent, not a helicopter, cop, or firefighter!

Because resiliency is linked to stronger decision-making skills and maturity, a brain drain is perfect for kids with ADHD. How can you help your kids to brain drain academic or social problems that your child, tween, or teen is currently tackling with mindfulness and resilience?

4. **Choosey Moms and Dads:** No, this is not a clichéd or old school peanut butter commercial, but I offer a tip to instill choices with kids of all ages to combat ADHD ramifications. When kids feel like they have some voice, power, choice, or control over situations, even something as small as using a pen or a pencil for a journal assignment, returning home by 10:00PM or 10:15 for curfew, or eating brown versus white rice for a family meal, they begin to invest in and embody more in resilience. Give choices and see what magic can happen in your household tonight!

5. **Thank You, Next:** Borrowed from Ariana Grande but without the singing chops and high ponytail action, I mindfully and deliberately try to steer kids with ADHD to purge themselves as prisoners of the past and truly see what's next with thanks and gratitude. By goal setting and planning in the now with kids, use questions to guide them toward finding resilience.

Because this technique can be boring, find fun and sensory-based ways like creative whiteboards or teen-friendly calendars to make this process more engaging. The old refrigerator technique for posting was too mundane for my creative teen niece, so I had to revert to organizational apps on her phone to do the trick after we had our heart to hearts in person.

6. **Effort Statements:** Because Chapter 10 discussed some communication techniques, I would also like to highlight the value of using effort statements. As noted, we often tend to focus on a child's weak areas and often do not find or take the time to positively and equitably acknowledge a child's, tween's, or teen's overall efforts throughout learning and social processes associated with ADHD.

In sum, it is time to think beyond grades and report cards. When kids with ADHD actually see that hard work and diligence are dually recognized by adults, they will likely be more apt to build and sustain resilience. Practice with effort statements that begin with "I notice," "I love how…" "I'm so impressed by your…" Find non-academic efforts, too, to balance the school-related, job, financial, or other ones, too. Mindfulness is truly all about finding balance and embracing the power in words.

7. **Giraffe It:** This tip means to use a growth mindset for kids, tweens, and teens with ADHD. Similar to the effort statements above, this technique is something that you want to lengthen or extend like a tall giraffe using positive encouragement and ways to keep your child focused on and reflective toward the growth and change process. What statements can you convey to show your child that he or she has exhibited strides and/ or progress socioemotionally, academically, or behaviorally? If your house feels like a zoo, *giraffe it* to channel serenity and resilience.

8. **Judge Judy or Jim**: Of course the blunt TV personality is definitely not what I am suggesting via this holistic method. Instead, I borrow from Dweck (2006) in *Mindset: The New Psychology of Success*, as the author emphasizes how learning from trial and error and directly from failure vividly teaches persistence, resilience, and strong character building traits. Forget the black robes and courtroom chaos; in essence, guide your kids to find and name the kernels of knowledge from struggles and

even failures. We call it our "makeover moments" in my house!

9. **Binoculars:** Parenting kids with ADHD often feels like one is operating with blinders. Dodge the blinders and don the binoculars with better resilience. While this strategy does not mean learning to hunt or bird watch, it is so helpful to teach kids to use invisible *binoculars* to observe mindfully, not overreact to adverse situations at home, with peers socially, or at work and school. This one works really well with my own daughter, the aspiring naturalist! Younger kids can also benefit from having a toy set to really ham it up!

10. **Family Night:** Kids also need to know that we're on their sides and teams unconditionally. Starting a ritual of a family night weekly or monthly, depending on your family's schedule, is so helpful since we are living in an era of very little face-to-face time.

During a family night, tap into family memories and create new ones with nostalgia. Play cards, board games, puzzles, charades, etc. Silber (2016) also suggests coloring together not only to bond and relax, but also to "clear their minds, and even cope with difficult emotions" (https://www.psychologytoday.com/us/articles/201609/what-s-the-deal-adult-coloring-books)? Break out that Scrabble or Twister, everyone!

Conclusion: A Complete Parenting Guide to Address ADHD: Mindful Approaches to Help Your Child, Tween, and Teen Improve Focus, Self-Regulation, and Success in School and Life

"True courage is in facing danger when you are afraid..."
— *L. Frank Baum, The Wonderful Wizard of Oz*

Just as Dorothy and her character family ultimately reached their final destination safely and successful with love, collaboration, resilience, and empowerment, I hope this book has also taught you how mindfulness can naturally address ADHD symptoms and proactively protect kids, tweens, teens, and families.

To sum the main objectives within this book as you navigate the *Yellow Brick Road* of ADHD holistically, I trust that this book clearly defined and traced the brief history of mindfulness for you. I also tried to unmask and rectify common ADHD stigmas and myths, so you can see beyond buzz words and trends to fully incorporate it with more confidence, accurate knowledge, and practical applications. Like the quote from Baum above, I also strongly applaud your courage, patience, passion, love, loyalty, and dedication to find new ways to connect with and empower your child.

While your kid with ADHD might not be a Hollywood Judy Garland or budding child prodigy, each child with ADHD is fully capable of fulfilling academic, socioemotional, behavioral, and vocational goals and dreams.

In brief, the book offered research, tips, and personal stories, so you can change gears from *stressed to impressed* as you hit cruise control on ADHD with Mindfulness for cultivating increased focus and improved self-regulation in your kids with ADHD. I have also included many techniques for attaining stress management in parents and kids with ADHD.

Just like Dorothy bravely battled the Wicked Witch of the West and her flying monkey brigade, you can collaboratively and positively guide your child with some mindfulness home strategies for more academic and vocational success, social skills, resilience, health, mindfulness, communicative effectiveness, and positive self-esteem. Similar to all the catchy songs and dances from *The Wizard of Oz* movie and musical versions, I also have added some ways to *move and groove* mindfully with physical strategies to cope with ADHD and some mood foods (and beverage ideas) to promote holistic eating for managing ADHD in your kitchens and homes. In general, many current studies exhibit how there is a clear mind, body, and soul link as far as a "patient's diet represents a modifiable target for improving mental health, and for some people, changing one's diet may improve ADHD symptoms" (Rucklidge, Taylor, & Johnstone, 2018, p. 15).

Please continue to revisit this book on your own journey toward achieving resilience in your family's work and success when coping with ADHD. As Wang & Adams (2016) posit in their book called *Bringing Mindfulness To Your Workplace*, a mindfulness approach to parenting embodies such a natural way to reduce stress, improve focus, extend memory, and promote morale. Even the most successful companies today such as Google, General Mills, and the *Huffington Post* have implemented mindfulness programs within their workplaces with diverse adults in every industry and location worldwide. These tactics truly work, and I can personally and professional vow for my work as a former educator and parent.

To further summarize and build upon the book's key points, Oaklander (2015) specifically cites how a new trial published in *Developmental Psychology* suggests that in kids with ADHD as young as 9, mindfulness vastly improved everything from social skills to math scores. Oaklander's (2015) research specifically uncovered how in the mindfulness classrooms, "the program incorporated sense-sharpening exercises like mindful smelling and mindful eating, along with cognitive mindfulness exercises like seeing an issue from another's point of view. Children did a three-minute meditation three times a day focusing on their breathing. They also acted on their lessons by practicing gratitude and doing kind things for others" (n.p.).

Regardless of how you utilize mindfulness to address ADHD with your own kids, tweens, and teens as a parent, family member, teacher, coach, mentor, neighbor, or professional, this book aspired to give you the wonderful wings to soar about labels and to labor with love and logic! I also tried to instill the knowledge that there is no one-stop-shop as far as quick ADHD cures. The bottom line and main takeaway that I want to end upon is borrowed directly from Yunus (2019) because it really does embody so much of what my book seeks to achieve as far as a mindfulness mindset: "there is not ONE right way to treat this complex condition. Often, ADHD is best managed by multiple modalities. Medication is one, behavior therapy is another, diet may be that added tool that can make a difference with your child today and in his/her future" (p. 26).

All in all, as Dorothy's courageous character constantly remarked throughout the marvelous movie to keep a positive vision, "There's no place like home!" This message is extremely relevant when discussing ways for parents to cope with kids who have ADHD. As Yunus (2019) also exclaims, "Setting our children up for the best adult life is part of our jobs as parents" (p. 26). I will end this book with full faith that you as the adults with take that steering wheel and guide your kids, tweens, and teens with ADHD in a mindful, peaceful, natural, and holistic direction to enable them to cruise with resilience and success as a result.